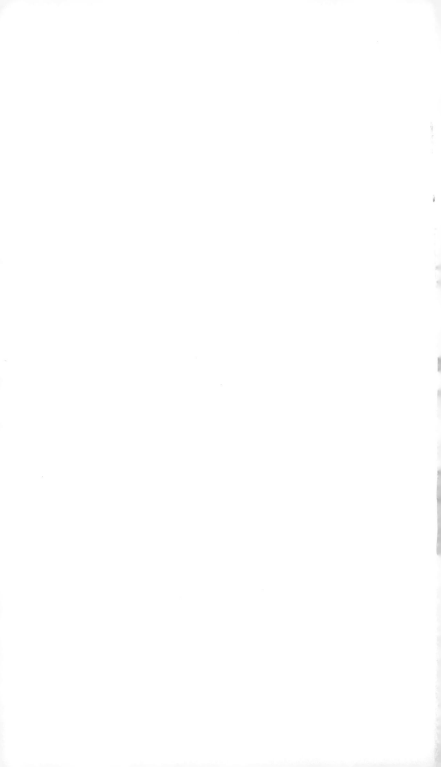

REIKI HEALING FOR BEGINNERS

The Ultimate Guide to Learn Mindfulness and Self-Healing Techniques. Mind Power Through Chakra Meditation, Increase Your Self-Esteem, Release Stress and Overcome Anxiety

© Spiritual Awakening Academy

Table of Contents

Introduction

Reiki healing allows you to connect with the energies of the Universe and use it in a way that encourages the body to heal itself. It can be used to treat aches and pains, overcome allergies and headaches, and even heal chronic or painful diseases. The results depend heavily on your abilities and your mindset, as it is important to be receptive to the Reiki energies for them to result.

Often, the emotional and physical health problems that we struggle with stem from blocked energy channels in the body. Energy channels can be blocked after certain life circumstances or from being neglected. As you learn to encourage the flow of Universal energy through your body, you can promote overall health and wellness. You can stop at learning to heal yourself or you can continue our practice to strengthen your abilities and possibly heal others.

Hopefully, this book has been able to help provide the foundation for Reiki knowledge that you can build upon later. For the time being, however, you should know what you need to put your Reiki skills to work. The only thing left to do is practice! Your abilities will strengthen with time and as you become more aware of the way that the energies of the universe and your body affect you.

The following chapters will discuss the process of Reiki and how you can get started with the great healing powers that come from it. Many people have never heard about Reiki before, but it is actually a powerful energy that is inside all of us. If you are dealing with chakras that are blocked up or energy that is not able to go freely through your body, using Reiki, either in person or over distance, can make all the difference.

This guidebook is going to spend some time talking about Reiki and the different parts that come with it. We will explore the fundamentals of what Reiki is all about and even how it relates to the chakras. We will also spend some time talking about how to perform Reiki on yourself, the training that a Reiki master has to go through, the benefits of using Reiki, and even some of the most common symbols for this practice. Once you give it a try using the information that is in this guidebook, you will be amazed at how much better you feel, emotionally, physically, and mentally.

When you are tired of dealing with emotional, mental or physical ailments and you have tried other methods that seem to have bad side effects or will make things worse, it may be time to give Reiki a try. Take some time to read through this guidebook and learn some of the basics of Reiki and how it can help you.

Chapter 1: Reiki Healing

Reiki is a form of therapy that promotes healing and balance in life.

The practice of Reiki improves relaxation and reduces stress, both of which are prevalent in society.

The focus of Reiki is to improve or increase the flow of positive energy through the use of energy that flows from the hands of the practitioner.

The idea is to improve areas of low or weak energy, which are considered areas of illness, to improve well being.

The word Reiki originates from the Japanese words for **Rei**, which refers to a "higher power" or "power of the universe", spirituality, or universal power, and **Ki**, which refers to energy or life force.

These two words combined are defined as a spiritually guided energy, which is the definition of Reiki.

The Origin of Reiki and How the Practice has Developed

The history of Reiki dates to ancient times, though the exact era or time period is unknown.

In more recent history, between the mid-1800s and early 20**th** century, the practice of Reiki was rediscovered and developed for modern use, as it is applied today.

Dr. Usai, a Buddhist monk from Japan, studied the ancient practice, discovering its benefits and developing Reiki further to enhance the benefits on a spiritual, mental and physical level.

In just over a century, Reiki is performed all over the world, from its roots in Japan to many countries across the globe, including western countries.

While many people may use Western-based medicine and treatments for a variety of illnesses and chronic conditions, many people also look towards Reiki and other forms of healing to strengthen their mind, body, and spirituality through this practice.

How does Reiki develop?

Reiki is developed through training sessions or classes, and a series of attunements.

There is a total of three levels of study in Reiki, which provides the foundation for understanding its healing energy and how it is applied as a therapy for yourself and others.

The power of Reiki develops over time, as it helps to clear and heal the mind, allowing a stronger flow of positive energy to transfer from one place or person to another.

For each level of Reiki, the student develops a deeper understanding and connection with universal energy.

With each attunement, there is a stronger enhancement of that connection, and while just one attunement can last for an indefinite length of time, some students choose to remain longer for each level, to deepen their experience and energy, either through more practice, additional attunements, or both.

Some people new to the practice, with little or no Reiki knowledge, may choose to take the first level only, for their own benefit or self-practice.

For others, the practice of Reiki is much more, and progressing to the third or master level is done with a great deal of passion and commitment.

Different Forms of Reiki

As Reiki developed over centuries, and within recent times, several forms of the practice became popular, and are known by their specific style or name.

While all forms of Reiki are essentially the same in principle, the style and methods in which it is practiced and treatment options used vary depending on the specific type. The following types are most commonly known as the following:

Jikiden Reiki

This is the most traditional and original form of Reiki practiced today.

It's also known as Eastern Reiki, as it is closely related to the way it was initially used when first developed.

This form has changed has not changed from its initial form and aims to closely follow the original model or techniques used in ancient times.

People who practice Jikiden Reiki are most interested in remaining with the traditional methods.

Jikiden is known as the purest form of Reiki, as it has changed the least in comparison to other forms. There are some distinct principles related to the traditional form of Reiki, known as Jikiden, including the following:

● It promotes the quick or accelerated healing process of surgical procedures and related medical techniques

● The healing process is spiritual, though it does not aim to change nor conflict with the different beliefs of other people.

In other words, it works regardless of your religion or faith. The focus is primarily on the level of energy that is channeled, which is universal and available to everyone.

● It aims to promote and heal the psychological side of addiction and related issues that stem from both psychological and physical foundations. This may include the alleviation of depression, anxiety, and forms of stress, which can be a recurring condition on their own or related to other conditions, which can also be treated in the same way.

● Another attribute of the goal of Jikiden Reiki is the ability to soothe and comfort without feeling invasive or uncomfortable, and this is also common in all forms of Reiki.

Hands are often placed over each area to be treated, or lightly touching the area for the same effect.

• This form of Reiki also aims to correct negative habits that are self-destructive, including compulsivity and addiction or repetitive behaviors that cause grief in our lives.

For example, people prone to substance abuse and gambling would benefit from this form of Reiki

Usui Reiki

Also known as the Western method, this style of Reiki remains close to Master Miao Usui's developments, though it has been revised and changed for common versions of the practice in Western countries.

Usui worked with the original form of Reiki, making some changes to enhance its ability, which has gone through further changes since.

Both forms (Jikiden and Usui), as with all Reiki styles, are referred to as a form of spiritual healing through physical means, where the light or energy is transferred or channeled through the hands from one person to the other, for the benefit of healing and other positive effects.

The Usui form of Reiki focuses on a specific set of principles and benefits as follows:

- There is a great deal of focus on accepting yourself as is and being able to practice and enjoy the benefits of Reiki anywhere at any time.

While the practice itself involves the transference of universal energy, there is a great deal of importance placed on the individual and their ability to benefit from this process.

- Like Jikiden Reiki, there is a focus on practicing in such a way that the experience is comfortable and brings a soothing sense to your mind and body.

- Usui is used as a way to help those who have passed away to transition or move from the current (or previous) physical existence to an afterlife or spiritual existence.

- There is a goal to reduce stress, including the tension and pressure that we accumulate daily, often without noticing.

Once this stress is lifted or calmed, the results are significant, and we feel lighter, and life becomes manageable and easier to face. Other benefits with the reduction of stress include less anxiety and a sense of fear.

- Also, like the Jikiden method, there is no conflict with other people's faiths or beliefs. The idea is to heal and comfort everyone, and this is a goal for all forms of Reiki.

- We all hide how we feel at some point, and some of us habitually hide our feelings and emotions like a regular way of dealing with them.

In Reiki, some of these emotions may rise to the surface, creating an experience that is liberating, though may cause some people to feel vulnerable. It's important to note that this is a natural effect of Reiki's strength in healing not only the physical but the emotional side as well.

- Usui Reiki aims to help people who have sustained injury and/or surgical procedures to heal quickly and effectively.

It also gives them the strength to endure the healing process and coping with life following the event.

- Sleep becomes easier and more qualitative after Reiki treatment.

Some people report the ability to fall asleep quicker than previously and experience a deeper, more satisfying rest than before.

- This form of Reiki is suitable for all ages and people, which is also the case with other forms of this practice.

Karuna Reiki

This is a form of Reiki that focuses on developing a deep sense of love and spreading it to others through the practice.

While the first two forms of Reiki focus on the physical healing process, along with the spiritual, Karuna Reiki aims to use more spiritual healing as a way to treat or improve others mentally and psychologically.

Some people who practice both Usui or Jikiden Reiki and Karuna, find that Karuna is overall stronger and has the potential for healing on a deeper level.

It builds upon the knowledge and sense of wisdom we already have, which helps us heal and improve faster on all levels (mentally, psychologically, physically, and spiritually).

The main idea is the extension of love and care to yourself and the people around you.

In doing this, the energy transfer is of a higher level and can promote healing more effectively as a result.

Many of the goals associated with this form of Reiki focus on emotional healing, and other conditions or issues associated with it:

● Karuna Reiki works to clear the mind of mental clutter and allow for better learning and a stronger understanding of knowledge.

This can help develop wisdom and promote a clearer understanding of our own thoughts and emotions.

● It provides a sense of relief and comfort for people suffering from loss or grief.

It allows them to cope while navigating through the stages of grief and processing the various emotions they will experience along this journey.

There is also some relief from the emotional pain that is experienced from a loss, and through other challenges in life as well.

- There is a focus on fostering a sense of self-acceptance and love and learning to accept the characteristics of ourselves that we find less appealing and ideal.

Some people are caught up in the negative aspects of what we don't like about our bodies and personalities, that we forget or lose sight of the positive. Karuna aims to help us accept that we are valuable despite our imperfections (or perceived imperfections), which helps boost self-esteem and a sense of worth.

- Personal goals are a focus of Karuna Reiki, and this works well with the sense of deep healing and emotional strength that is fostered through this practice.

In accepting who we are and improving our own self-love, we become more capable of achieving our own personal goals, as well as work and professional milestones.

Other benefits of Karuna Reiki include further development of self-reliance and less codependency.

The overall focus on this form of Reiki is to alleviate and treat a lot of emotional disorders and inconsistencies that we all face from time to time.

For some people, this can be more challenging to treat than others, though over time, there is a great deal of improvement and confidence as a result.

Couples looking to improve their relationship and communication skills with one another, as well as with others in their lives, can benefit significantly from Karuna Reiki.

This practice works well with both Western forms of therapy (therapy and Western medicine) as well as other alternative forms for medicine or wellness.

Sekehem Reiki (also known as Sichim Reiki)

This form of Reiki is based in Egypt and is considered the extension of healing and well being from the Egyptian Goddess Sekhmet.

The form of energy used or channeled is considered vibrational and full of light, which rejects all forms of negativity and pain that are associated with it.

The main principle of this form of Reiki is to promote positivity and build a stronger sense of spirituality through the opening of chakras and delivering a strong light or healing power.

There is a renewed sense of balance and contentment with this treatment, which begins gradually, and increases to an intense level.

The effects are powerful, and many people report the effects of just one session lasting for more than several days.

Sekehem or Sichim Reiki is often used with essential oils.

The treatment focuses on healing, emotionally and mentally, from situations that cause grieving or other stressful scenarios, including marital breakdown, loss of employment and other difficult experiences in life.

One of the main effects noticed by people who receive this form of Reiki as a treatment is the draining of energy from the negative, and a sense of relief or peace that follows.

The feelings can be intense, though favorable, and soothing at once.

The main benefits of this Reiki are as follows:

- A deeper sense of awareness and focus in life. A sense of purpose is stronger, and this fosters a better sense of confidence as well.

- Promoting connections between other people in our lives and our relationships with them. Treatment can provide an opportunity to deepen these ties and help us appreciate the positive connections we have with the closest people to us.

- The deep sense of enlightenment and spirituality, including a stronger sense of inner peace and acceptance.

- Stronger and faster healing of the emotional, spiritual, and physical within ourselves.

Karuna Reiki is a powerful way to connect with nature and the universe on a spiritual level while improving our own state of well being in the process.

The growing intensity and long-lasting effects of this practice create a long-lasting effect that can be transferred to others as it benefits us, either as a practitioner, a client, or a student.

Lightarian Reiki
This form of Reiki both combines and expands the purpose of Usui and Karuna forms, focusing on a deep

sense of loving energy with strong self-building goals and healing properties.

Reiki Masters practice Lightarian Reiki to improve their spiritual level and increase their level beyond, to promote stronger healing abilities by channeling more vibrational forms of energy.

There are different bands or levels of energy in Reiki, eight in total, which create a path to higher awareness and spirituality.

The Usui and Karuna forms of Reiki are concentrated with the first two bands, while the remaining six are reached through Lightarian Reiki, to connect with Ascended Masters or a higher sense of being.

During this process of moving through the different bands of energy, there is a growing sense of empowerment within, which helps create stronger sources of energy during practice on others as well as for yourself personally.

What are the main properties and benefits of Lightarian Reiki?

The following advantages can be gained through the process of Reiki meditation and self-practice, which is detailed further in this book:

- As you progress through the higher forms of energy, this will benefit clients in your practice. You'll be giving or channeling a higher form of energy for faster and stronger healing ability.

- Along with helping others, you'll notice a higher sense of personal peace and healing within.

- Growing sensitivity and awareness for further spiritual development.

All forms of Reiki are powerful and create strong channels of energy for healing and self-betterment in many ways.

The most popular form of Reiki practiced today is Usui, as his methods are easy to follow and readily practiced throughout North America.

This form of practice remains mostly traditional, with aspects of Master Usui's enhancements, which were implemented around one hundred years ago.

If you are interested in exploring other forms of Reiki in practice, a Master or instructor may be able to refer additional resources or materials to study different forms, or depending on their own experience and training; they may be able to offer helpful advice as well.

Chapter 2: Reiki Healing Techniques

Karuna Reiki

Karuna is a word that means any action that helps to diminish other people's suffering. In Sanskrit, Karuna means "compassionate action." The Karuna system of Reiki is a technique developed by William L. Rand when he used the symbols channeled by other Reiki Masters like Kellie-Ray Marine, Pat Courtney, Marla Abraham, and Marcy Miller. Rand found the symbols to be very valuable, but he felt that they still had a lot of potential locked deep within them. He used guided meditation to become attuned with the symbols to unlock their full potential, and he called this new Reiki technique Karuna.

Karuna Reiki's energy is applied with more focus and also works on all energy bodies simultaneously. People who receive attunement from their Reiki teacher only when they have become qualified Reiki practitioners. They often need to report to their Spirit Guides, Angels, and their Higher Self, and then afterwards they feel their presences at times.

Benefits of Karuna Reiki

- Non-invasive

- Helps heal unconscious patterns/habits

- Can help with sleeping problems

- Can help easy panic attacks, fatigue, and muscle pain

- Can help with the manifestation of personal goals

- Helps pull out the negative energy, or blockages in your ki flow and helps release pain

- Can also help ease emotional pain

- Does not require you to convert into another religion

- Heals the body on a cellular level

- Helps you deal with past-life issues

- Helps you fix communication problems

- Helps you deal with co-dependency

- Helps mend relationships and makes them better

- Helps you be more mindful and in the moment

- Helps you shatter your denial habits

- Helps with self-image problems\

- Improves learning and promote clarity of the mind

Sekhem or Seichim Reiki

Sekhem is an ancient Egyptian word that means "Universal Energy or Power", roughly translate as "Power of Powers". Sekhem in Egyptian hieroglyphs is symbolized by the scepter, and it represents the connection between Heaven and Earth.

Sekhem healing energy can help accelerate your spiritual growth, but most importantly, it can open communication channels with your "higher self" and with the "All That Is", which can mean different things to different faiths (the Cosmic Universe, the Divine Creator, the Soul of Souls, etc.) There are no other known energy system that can compare with the high vibrational energy of Sekhem, nor does any other energy work at a deeper soul level.

Sekhem Reiki promotes being more responsible for your life. It also allows you to heal, and it helps your personality and spirituality, so you can find your soul's purpose and unlock your full potential.

Benefits of Sekhem or Seichim Reiki

- Fast physical, spiritual, and emotional healing

- Quickens the never ending process of spiritual development and enlightenment

- Assists in the manifestation of goals

- Improves your "inner sight" and your ability to sense the energy around you

- Increases your "feeling of being alive" by making you more aware of the present

- Increases your self-awareness and your relationships with others

Western Reiki

Almost all of the Reiki practiced in Japan is Westernized Reiki, which is quite ironic considering that Reiki originated from Japan. There was a time when people thought that there were no more any legitimate Reiki practitioners left in Japan. That is why when Reiki was reintroduced into the country, the Japanese people who wished to learn it had to visit North America to get tutelage. However, the successors of Usui-sensei have always been in Japan.

There are also the surviving students of Chujiro Hayashi, which was one of the prominent students of Mikao Usui. One of his students was Hawayo Takata, who was believed to be the person who introduced Reiki to the Western hemisphere.

Benefits of Western Reiki

- Promotes acceptance of oneself

- Can help minimize pain and discomfort; can actually be used to aid in natural childbirth

- Can assist a dying person's soul transcend peacefully to the afterlife

- Can aid in being more mindful of one's thoughts and physical feelings

- Can help uncover hidden emotions so they can be easily healed

- Can balance the chakras in the body

- Can be used to complement other medical treatments safely

- No need to convert to other religions

- Non-invasive and gentle healing

- Provides natural pain relief

- Promotes deep relaxation and helps cure sleeping disorders

- Promotes wholistic health and well-being

- Is safe for use by pregnant women

- Hastens the recovery from surgery sickness, and eases labor pains

- Can help ease and eliminate stress

Chapter 3: Benefits of Reiki

Increased Ability to Deal with Negative Energies and Stresses of the World

The benefit of Reiki is that it helps relieve the weight of any negative experiences you may have. As you walk through your office building or down the street, you will notice a new recognition for those things that do not serve your purpose. You will understand what things do not serve your purpose in life and which encounters leave you in an undesirable mental state. Then, you can learn to block the energies from things you do not want to experience and avoid those situations that you can, should they not promote the satisfied, energized feeling that you should feel.

Ability to Heal Others

If you decide to progress past the point of Reiki healing for yourself, it is easy to become attuned with the world and direct your energy in a way that corrects the energy flow of others. As you choose people to practice with, it is important to choose those that are opened to the idea of Reiki healing. You may find yourself put off of the practice altogether if you try it on a relative with health problems who does not have an open mind to new age topics like Reiki. Keep in mind that it is not always your failure. Reiki will not work on someone who cannot open their mind and body to the flow of energy.

Physical Healing

Physical healing is one of the benefits of Reiki that people seem to be most skeptical about. They do not understand how something that restores energy can help relieve the symptoms of their physical condition, whether it is a simple headache or a chronic illness. Those who doubt this method have often been healed using a Western form of medicine, which commonly focuses on treating the ailment directly instead of using a full-body approach.

This is one of the reasons that people turn to alternative or holistic medicine when a more scientific approach has healed them. In many cases, the results have been a complete turnaround. There are even anecdotes of people who have turned to Reiki healing and other alternative medicines and had success in healing cancer, relieving chronic pain, and fighting off severe illness.

Mental and Emotional Healing

People's pain and sickness are not always visible. Many people struggle with anxiety, depression, repressed emotions, and other mental and emotional states. They may not even be aware of their emotional state or what is causing it. Reiki does not always help you heal emotions unless you deal with them; however, it can make you more aware of your emotional state.

This awareness can help you understand your problems. It can also help you tap into the divine nature and understand your purpose in life. As you continue to connect to the energy that exists within everything and all around you, it can help cultivate more positive emotions in your life, including connectedness, love, intimacy, kindness, compassion, and sharing.

Increased Spirituality

The flow of energy that you experience with Reiki can help you notice the interconnectedness between all the life forms of earth. As you connect to all that is living around you, you will feel a greater connection to the divine. You will also feel as if you are part of something greater than what exists in your immediate world. For many people, this creates the feeling of being connected to something great and powerful. It offers reassurance that you are present in the universe and you know that you are loved by and connected to the spiritual beings, both living and non-living that you may encounter through your day.

Greater Compassion

The connectedness that you feel when regularly cleansing and connecting to your internal source of energy can help you find greater compassion for all that exists in the world. You will be more compassionate and empathetic when you encounter others who are in pain, whether emotional or physical. You will also be more tolerant and understanding of others, aware that you cannot possibly understand their specific situation. As you learn this deep compassion for others, you will also learn to be kinder to and have greater compassion for yourself. This can help heal people who struggle with emotional trauma or low self-esteem, as they often struggle with treating themselves as well as they would treat others.

Stress Relief

Stress relief is a major benefit of Reiki, as it is responsible for many of its effects. When you regularly relax and provide yourself with stress relief, it gives your body and mind a much-needed break from the fast-paced world around you. This stress relief can help you sleep better at night and promotes a stronger immune system since your body is getting the support that it needs to be healthy. This can also reduce blood pressure.

Detoxifies the Body and Mind

A major part of the Reiki process is the removal of
negative energies and toxins from your body. It
cleanses the body and helps you naturally eliminate
toxins that may have built up in your organs, digestive
system, and bloodstream. You naturally encounter
these toxins through your day—they are in some of
the foods that you eat and the air that you breathe.
Reiki also detoxifies the mind, clearing it of blockages
that are stopping you from dealing with emotional
trauma. This clearer state of mind and deeper
understanding help you on the path to healing.

Energizing and Rejuvenating

Reiki is a very energizing practice. As you tap into
your spiritual energy and the connectedness between
you and all that is in the universe, you will feel your
energy grow. You will feel reinvigorated as the life
force flows through your body. Some Reiki experts
also say that the rejuvenation from Reiki can postpone
that aging process and promote overall vitality.

Balance and Harmony

Reiki is a non-invasive technique of healing that
promotes your overall wellbeing by working along
with your body's natural ability to heal itself. Reiki
does not just promote your overall wellbeing but it
also helps re-energize and revitalize your body. It

brings about a sense of balance, not only to your physical body but your spiritual and mental aspects of life as well. It is an energy healing system that doesn't provide superficial solutions but helps deal with the primary cause of any troubles in your life. By practicing Reiki, you can easily restore your mental and emotional balance.

Energy and Balance

For your overall wellbeing, it is essential that your body, mind, and soul are in harmony. Reiki allows you to get rid of any blocks of energy within and promotes your overall balance. By using Reiki healing regularly, you can become calmer and at peace. It is a great way to deal with stress. Apart from this, it also improves your cognitive abilities. Once your mind is clear and free from stress, your ability to learn and retain information also enhances.

Apart from this, it also helps and emotional healing. If you have frequent mood swings, then Reiki can help reverse this process. Strengthening and healing your relationships can also be possible through this. Your ability to love others and receive love from others dramatically improves when you start using Reiki. This helps strengthen your ability to form and maintain relationships.

Relaxation and Stress Relief

If you want to let go of unnecessary stress and tension from your body, then Reiki is the answer. While using Reiki healing, you don't consciously have to do anything; you merely need to allow the energy from this healing process to remove any tension from your body and mind. You will start to feel lighter and more relaxed from within. Apart from this, it also increases your awareness of the state of your mind and body.

Once you are aware of what you feel and how you feel or why you feel the way you feel, it becomes easier to manage your emotions. You get an opportunity to learn to be more attuned to your body's needs and your emotional wellbeing. It helps you assess the inner wisdom and knowledge that exists within you.

Pain Relief

Reiki helps alleviate pain while improving your physical health. By correcting any imbalances of energy in your body, it improves your physical health and enables your body to function optimally. It is a non-invasive healing process and can provide relief from arthritis, migraines, or any other physical ailments. Apart from this, it is also used to alleviate symptoms of asthma, menopause, and insomnia.

Better Focus

Reiki can make you feel centered and grounded. This helps improve your focus and provides mental clarity. Most of us often focus on our past or worrying about the future. Dwelling in thoughts associated with either of these is not going to do you much good in your present. Reiki helps you live in the present moment. It improves your ability to accept things that come your way and work your way through challenging circumstances. Instead of reacting, you can learn to respond.

Natural Detoxification

Reiki enables the natural detoxification of your body and improves the functioning of your immune system. The modern lifestyle is full of stress, which triggers your body's fight or flight response. Reiki shifts your body from the fight or flight mode towards the rest, and it starts to behave and act like it is supposed to. This state doesn't symbolize non-productivity or inactivity. It merely improves your sleep cycle based on the circadian rhythm. It essentially improves your sleep cycle along with the functioning of your digestive system. These two things are essential for your optimal health and vitality. If your body starts functioning healthy, and you get the rest you deserve, your productivity will improve.

Improved Sleep

Perhaps the most obvious outcome of a Reiki session is relaxation. Once your body and mind are both relaxed, your ability to sleep peacefully through the night will improve. Once you get good quality, undisturbed sleep, you will feel more energized in the morning.

Self-Healing

Reiki works along with your body's metabolism and accelerates its ability to heal itself. It helps restore the natural state of your body and encourages it to perform the way supposed to. From your blood pressure to your heart rate, you will notice an improvement in all aspects of your health. Once you start practicing Reiki on yourself, the way you breathe also improves. Most of us are not conscious of the way we breathe. Usually, taking slow and deep breaths is recommended because it helps with better absorption and transportation of oxygen in the body. By becoming conscious of your breathing, you can improve your mental clarity. This is essential because of all the oxygen that boosts your brain and improves your cognitive functions.

Emotional Cleansing

Reiki not only helps improve your physical health but it also helps your spiritual and emotional wellbeing.

You needn't necessarily be spiritual to enjoy the benefits of Reiki. However, if you are interested in reconnecting with your spiritual side and improve your emotional health, then Reiki will come in handy. Reiki doesn't just target a specific symptom but it addresses all the aspects related to your overall health. Perhaps this is one of the reasons why it can bring about certain shifts to the flow of energy in your body. Once any energy imbalances removed from your body, your body performs the way it was intended to. This gives you better clarity and increases your ability to stay in the moment. These factors help process your emotions and handle them in a better way. All in all, it helps emotional cleansing.

Alternate Treatments

Reiki is often used as a complementary therapy along with conventional medicines because it promotes relaxation of your body and mind. When you are relaxed, your body's ability to heal itself improves. It also accelerates the healing benefits of any conventional therapy. Reiki helps you sleep better and attain mental peace. Since it is non-invasive and can be administered gently, it works amazingly well with other therapies and medical treatments. Reiki can be provided without physically touching the recipient's body; this works especially well if the recipient is suffering from any severe injuries like burns.

Another benefit of Reiki is that you can practice Reiki on yourself. You don't have to go to a Reiki practitioner to get Reiki. Once you learn this healing technique, you can start practicing yourself or even provide Reiki for others.

Chapter 4: Symbols of Reiki

As you learn more and more about Reiki, you will come across different symbols. You have likely seen similar ones in other methods, considering you may have seen Kanji in Japanese language. In Reiki healing, there are five traditional symbols.

Introduced as part of the Reiki system back in 1922, Dr. Mikao Usui envisioned the symbols at the end of his 21-day fast. It has also been said that their origins are much older since they have already been a part of the world while Dr. Usui was still studying what Reiki would become. Since then, the symbols have become essential tools in the world of Reiki healing.

5 Traditional Reiki Symbols

When you aim to master Reiki, it is important to remember the five symbols that have been deemed traditional. These symbols represent the different aspects of Reiki, as well as how they can help you in your journey. They are seen as the keys that will open the doors to higher levels of awareness. As such, they are considered sacred and holy. In the olden times, they were not shared with the public. Nowadays, the symbols can be seen by everyone.

As you learn more about these symbols, take note that they do not hold any special powers. They function more as guiding tools for students and masters so that they can focus on the energy that they hold within. They are also part of the Reiki's energy presence.

Power

The "power" symbol, also known as cho ku rei, represents the increase and decrease of one's power. It is displayed as a coil and believed to be the regulator of the energy when it expands and contracts. Its intention is the light switch. Depending on where it is drawn, the power symbol can show the users its ability to enlighten or illuminate them on a spiritual level.

Harmony

The "harmony" symbol's intention is purification. Also known as the sei hi ki, it is used as a way towards mental and emotional healing. The harmony symbol is represented as a bird's wing dashing or the wave flowing across the ocean.

Distance

The "distance" symbol, which is known as hon sha ze sha, represents the intention for timelessness. It is displayed as a tower called a pagoda. Used as a way to send energy across distances, it symbolizes someone's ability to share their qi even when the ones they are sharing it with are not in the same physical plane.

Master

The "master" symbol, also known as dai ko myo, represents everything about Reiki. The symbol is displayed as a combination of multiple symbols and shows the users who have ascended their levels to finally become the masters. They share not only what they have learned but also heal when they are initiating attunements.

Completion

The "completion" symbol, also known as raku, represents the intention for closure. The symbol is displayed as a lightning bolt. As soon as the attunement is done, the users can now reach the completion of their ascending journey when they finally see this symbol.

How Symbols Are Used

Now that you have learned what the symbols are and what they mean, you have to know how they are used in Reiki.

Power Symbol

For the power symbol, it can serve as a catalyst for various purposes, such as purification and physical cleansing. It is also a useful tool for someone to increase their attention and focus. But most of all, it is commonly used when beginning a Reiki healing session to boost the practitioner's power. A good way to see how the power symbol works is when you are healing injuries. When you manage to cultivate the power symbol, it will be able to alleviate someone's pain and treat all light and major injuries.

The power symbol can also be used when one has the intention to get rid of negative energy. After all, it symbolizes purification, so you can expect to feel more positive energy when you make good use of the power symbol. This means that relationships, fortunes, and karma can all be purified with the help of the power you will get from the latter.

Harmony Symbol

For the harmony symbol, it can be used as a way for people to recover from traumas and past events that affect them. Practitioners use it when treating addictions and depression and unblocking creative energies.

The harmony symbol can also help you achieve focus and retain information that you are trying to learn from various resources. For instance, if you want to remember all the things that you have read in a book or the Reiki moves without having to refer to too many resources, the harmony symbol is there to help you out.

As stated earlier, the harmony symbol works when you treat addictions. So, you can kick the old habits and cultivate better ones as this symbol helps you see yourself in a much better light.

Distance Symbol

Practitioners use the distance symbol to help people go through their personal issues. For example, when a person has an identity issue, it can guide them to be more comfortable with others even when they are not in the same room. It can also be used to bring energy from great distances. Though the receiver and the sender are not in the same physical plane, they can still feel each other through the spiritual plane.

Nevertheless, take note that the distance symbol must be used correctly in order for it to work. You won't get much out of it if you do not use it properly.

Master Symbol

For the master symbol, it is used to gain enlightenment. This comes in handy especially when Reiki masters are administering attunement to people who wish to become practitioners and ascend through its levels. Self-healers can also use the symbol to know how they can combine the powers of the other symbols.

The master symbol is considered as an important one among the five traditional Reiki symbols because aside from the benefits described above, it is helpful when you are doing Reiki meditation, strengthening your intrapersonal relationship, improving your immune system, and healing your physical body

Completion Symbol

Finally, the completion symbol is used to bring closure and rise with the awakened energy. It represents the ascension of a person from being a mere student to becoming a master. They feel a new kind of energy flow within themselves, which is something that they have never experienced in the previous levels.

You can utilize this symbol when you are about to end your Reiki session. You can draw or visualize the completion symbol and know that you have finally completed what needed to be done throughout the session.

The symbols are used by putting them on materials that can help the Reiki practitioners remember them while performing healing sessions. For example, someone can print them on posters while others can hang small tags as decorations. This is a way to let everyone know that the symbols are all around them so that they can achieve their goals and purpose with each session.

Still, do not think the Reiki symbols are used one at a time. You can actually use two or more at a time or even combine the symbols' powers to perform a variety of healing methods that others do not offer. An example of this is when you are sending Reiki for an upcoming event that's important in your life. By mixing up the beneficial symbols, you will be able to feel more focused and enlightened when the time is about to come.

Another example is when you try to heal someone from a distance. They might feel some kind of emotional turmoil or grief, to be specific. You can then combine the symbols' powers by holding an item that gives you a strong connection to the person. You will draw or visualize the symbols so that when you perform the healing process, you can send the Reiki energy and let the person know that you are doing it all with a strong and good intention.

In this day and age, you can also integrate the symbols in your life by putting them on your technological devices. This way, when something is amiss, you can check your gadget to see the symbols and remember that things will be alright. So, if your day is not going well or you just need a little breather, have a look at the symbols, remember why you are doing what you are doing, and tread on.

With the traditional Reiki symbols at your disposal, you can use them as you learn to master Reiki.

Chapter 5: Reiki And The Chakras

Reiki is chakra work. That is, we work on the seven main energy centers that lie along the spine in the subtle body. Via the crown or crown chakra, we absorb light energy. This energy then flows from top to bottom through one center after another and is transformed in each chakra so that it can be used for our physical level - organs, glands. Finally, at the root center, it unites with the earth energy that we constantly absorb through the soles of our feet.

Chakras are not static points, but moving light wheels - as their name implies (the Sanskrit word chakra means "wheel"). They are dynamic or rotating centers that distribute light energy in all directions, like small suns. The movement is created by the life energy that flows into the respective chakra and brings it to life. When the life force is in flux, the chakras begin to vibrate and bloom. The more life force flows through them, the more beautiful they bloom, and this is visible in our charisma.

"Thou shalt acquire riches in the heavens, not on earth," says the Bible. We do this by working with Reiki and other types of meditation on our charisma.

What we achieve in this way remains with us. If it were part of the physical body, it would be lost with death and we would have to start all over again, but this progress is not part of the physical body but is stored in the etheric body.

With the authentic Reiki, we bring about a harmonious development of our energy centers. The chakras, which are not as advanced as others, evolve over time and flourish. You can really visualize this as the blossoming of a flower bud in the sunlight: we are becoming more and more permeable to the light energy and the flow of life energy within us is getting stronger. It all happens in a gentle way. The universal energy activated in the attunements is always harmless and supportive and always depends on the real needs of the recipient. Overstraining or "too much" is thus excluded.

All degrees of authentic Reiki develop all seven chakras, but the emphasis is always on the energy center associated with the corresponding degree. In the first degree, especially the root or base center is activated. We lose our existential fears and get a positive relationship to responsibility and matter. The second degree emphasizes the sacral chakra, the seat of sensuality, sexuality, creativity, and reproduction.

Little by little, we recognize our divine potential and live it. In the third degree, above all, the solar network is activated, the seat of our self-confidence and our self-esteem. The fourth degree has a special relation to the heart chakra, the chakra of love. By developing this center, we develop our humanity and can feel, love, cry, laugh, share, empathize and pray. We become love. Doubt and suspicion disappear as well as hairiness and too much disinterestedness. Instead, trust floods the heart. In deep meditation or in Reiki you are connected to the whole of creation, from heart to heart, beyond mind and language.

In the fifth degree, especially the connection between heart and neck is strengthened. Our love becomes more meditative. We feel the desire to share love with each other. With the sixth degree, which especially activates the third eye, our consciousness is increasingly developing in the direction of: "I am love." When the energy in the sixth chakra is awakened, it is experienced as a tremendous expansion, as a possibility, a glimpse to throw cosmic or infinite.

When the energy flows freely in the seventh or crown chakra, we finally arrive home. A waking crown chakra corresponds to the seventh day of creation on which the Creator rests. There is nothing left to do.

Only now that we have become masters of ourselves can we really help others. It is also called "Unio Mystica," the mystical union of yin and yang. Only at this highest summit of synthesis is true, lasting fulfillment possible.

However, it's less about knowing about the chakras than about feeling them authentic. Working on the chakras - and this is Reiki - serves to dissolve energy blockages. When in the end all seven chakras have become so active that they merge into a single pillar of light, it is called enlightenment.

The Benefits of a Balanced Chakra System

Throughout our lives we are put into situations that cause us physical trauma or distress, emotional instability, and leave us mentally drained and spiritually stunted. This can put a stop to your life. Feeling this way could also make your push your friends and family away. All of this can lead to a downward spiral where you feel lost, as if you don't know who you are anymore and you don't know why this is happening to you. One of the reasons that you feel like this could be because one or more of your chakras is unbalanced.

When one or more of our chakras is blocked, then energy cannot freely flow through us. Often when a chakra within us is blocked, a part of our life is left blocked as well. This can lead to many unhealthy and bad effects to our minds, bodies, and souls. This is why it's important to unblock and balance your chakra system. Remember that your chakras are like pools of water in your body and they are all connected and flow through each other, so even if only one of your chakras is blocked it will throw all of the chakras out of balance and start affecting you.

Besides feeling happier, healthier and more in tune with yourself and the universe there are many benefits to balancing your chakra system. Each chakra is blocked by a specific thing and each chakra brings something to your life if they are balanced. Here I will describe the overall benefits you will achieve when you have all seven chakras balanced.

Amazing Benefits of Balanced Chakras:

1. Unblocking your chakras will also release blocked emotional and physical energy. Blocked emotional energy could lead to unresolved feelings of sadness or vulnerability. Unblocking this energy will make you feel happier, more energetic, and less vulnerable.

2. Blocked chakras can lead to confusion and difficulty with understanding simple tasks and solving problems. Unblocking your chakras will leave you feeling more motivated and confident. You'll be more likely to succeed in all your endeavors and reach your goals.

3. With unblocked chakras you will feel and look younger, and you will feel healthier than ever before.

4. You will feel more in touch with your intuition. Blocked chakras can make you doubt yourself and feel negative about your thoughts and feelings. With balanced chakras you will trust your intuition more and no longer doubt yourself.

5. You will feel a stronger emotional connection in your relationships. Having balanced chakras allows you to be more in touch with your emotions which will let you feel things more deeply. Although you will be more connected with your emotions, you will be in full control so you won't be overwhelmed by them. Having a balanced chakra system is just one step towards fully controlling your emotional state and being able to connect to others' emotions in relationships.

6. Lying is something we all do. Whether it's to save ourselves from embarrassment or save someone else from being hurt. However, if your chakras are balanced, you will be able to understand the importance of the truth better and you will be able to express the truth easier. You will also be more understanding when hearing the truth from others, even if it is a hard, cold truth.

7. You will be more comfortable and self-confident. It's no secret that we all feel a little insecure in our own skin. Having a balanced chakra system can fill you with confidence and help you be more comfortable with yourself and even with your own sexuality.

8. Balancing your chakras can even lead you to have a better memory.

9. A balanced chakra system can give you more energy and motivation. This can help you with weight loss among other things.

10. Balancing your chakras can help you connect to your subconscious mind. This has many benefits on its own, along with feeling more aware.

11. Balancing your chakras can help you rid your life of many things that plague us all: stress, anxiety, insomnia, depression, addiction, and so on. Having a balanced chakra system means having a balanced life.

12. Having a balanced chakra system will allow you to think more clearly and will even promote creativity.

13. You will have more mental toughness. This means that you will be able to withstand more abuse and hurt from the world. The world can be harsh and any number of things can leave us feeling hurt and broken. Having a balanced chakra system will allow you to be able to withstand the world's harsh ways and will leave you feeling more capable to fight against or ignore it.

14. With balanced chakras your overall health will improve and your immune system will be more capable of fighting back against illness. When your body is in harmony you are healthy and strong. When your body is disorganized and unbalanced you are left weak and open to illness. If you balance your chakras and your body then you will be healthy and stay healthy.

These are simple benefits that come from a balanced chakra system but they can lead to you feeling like a new person. You will feel like you can do and handle anything life throws at you. There are many things we do in modern times that we weren't meant to do. We weren't meant to sit in an office all day long and work. We aren't supposed to be stressing about a hundred different things all at once. We weren't meant to spend our lives working in order to survive. This is why so many people live with unbalanced chakras. This is why so many people today are sick and tired all the time.

There are so many parts of the modern world that can lead to our chakras being blocked and unbalanced. The modern world is designed to unbalance us. We can fight back by putting ourselves first and focusing on balancing our chakras. Once your chakras are balanced you will be more equipped to handle the things in life that are set to unbalance us.

Negative Energy versus Positive Energy

What exactly unbalances our chakras? The answer is simple; negative energy.

The universe is filled with energy, both negative and positive. Energy from the universe flows into us. The positive energy flows through us freely but the negative energy cannot flow as easily. It is more likely to become stuck inside of us if we do not know how to release it properly. When the negative energy starts to pile up, that is when the natural flow of positive energy is stopped and our chakras are blocked.

The differences between positive energy and negative energy are many. However, the main difference between the two is how each of them enters our bodies. Once again, the universe is filled with energy but our bodies willingly let the positive energy in. We do not willingly let the negative energy into our bodies. The negative energy forces its way into our bodies through certain events.

Negative energy thrives in traumatic experiences, emotional hurt and mental challenges. Things like pain, whether it's physical or emotional, invite negative energy into our bodies. Stress, anxiety, self-doubt, hatred, anger, depression, addiction, loathing, and jealousy are all part of the flow of negative energy. These are the things that invite negative energy into our bodies and the negative energy becomes stuck inside our energy pools if we don't have the tools or knowledge to release it properly.

We are not all born with the ability to properly release negative energy from our bodies. Things like traumatic life experiences are difficult to live through and even more difficult to let go of. Something as simple as being yelled at by your parents for breaking a dish can send negative energy into your body. When we were children, we didn't know how to properly understand and release this negative energy. Chances are that that negative energy is still inside of you. This is how easily our chakras can become blocked by negative energy. The more it builds up, the worse it can be for your health and the harder it will be to release it.

Although this knowledge may seem overwhelming and it may make you feel hopeless, there is still a reason to have hope. We are all born with the ability to take in positive energy from the universe and give positive energy back to the universe. Understanding, identifying, and releasing negative energy is something we need to learn. Identifying the negative energy is always the first step. Now that you know what negative energy is and where it comes from, you are already on your way to learning how to release it properly and unblock your chakras. Once you learn to release the negative energy inside you and your chakras are balanced, you will see that it is not as easy for the negative energy to enter your body as it was before.

With Balanced Chakras Comes a Balanced Life

We all want to feel balanced in life. We want to know that we have a purpose in life or that we are walking the path that is meant for us. Having a balanced life may seem like a far-fetched idea but it's never too far out of our reach. Living a balanced life is all about having balanced chakras.

We are living in a world that we are not supposed to be living in. The modern life of technology and pollution is not the life that was intended for us. It is an unnatural existence. This is why most of us live our lives with unbalanced chakras and unhealthy bodies. Our bodies are more prone to illness and injury when the energy inside us isn't flowing the way it should be.

When you think about it, everything is energy. We are made up of energy, everything is made up of energy. The best way to live life is to be able to tell the good energy from the bad energy and learning to accept the good energy into our bodies while expelling the bad energy.

Our chakras are ponds of energy and they are being fed by a waterfall of positive energy from the universe. All of the ponds are connected. All of our chakras are connected. If one is blocked by negative energy then the natural flow of energy inside us is disrupted and it affects our health. We must not only pay more attention to ourselves but we must pay more attention to all of our chakras.

If we wish to have a healthy and balanced life then our minds, bodies, souls, and chakras must also be in perfect balance.

Chapter 6: Levels of Reiki

Before getting started with Reiki, it is important to know that it comes in different levels or degrees. They can be seen as rankings, much like how an employee can go from a low-level position to a high-level one in their respective field. You can also see them as a way for an individual to upgrade their skills, going from beginner to intermediate until reaching the advanced level.

3 Levels or Degrees of Reiki

In the world of Reiki, there are three levels or degrees. When one is interested in practicing Reiki, you will need to climb these levels to master the healing methods. They will especially come in handy when you want to see what goes beyond the current level you are in. Such degrees also represent a person's ability to fully understand Reiki healing. This is a way for the student to become a master in the end.

First Degree

The first degree or Level 1 of Reiki is a practitioner's initiation. It is open to everyone and has the goal of helping individuals to be comfortable with the Reiki principles. This is where you will learn the ins and outs of the practice, as well as how it works right from the start.

The students who wish to become practitioners in the near future will have their attunement in Level 1. Done by the Reiki masters, the attunement will help them connect to the life energy that surrounds us.

Also, it is known that students going through Level 1 will be given lessons about Reiki's history and methods along with group practice sessions.

In a way, the first degree encourages practitioners to take the first step towards mastery.

Second Degree

The second degree or Level 2 allows you to practice Reiki on others while making use of the symbols and slowly expanding or opening more energy channels. This is where the student will begin to apply what they have learned from Level 1 and share their energy to others. They can also understand what the symbols mean and how they can be utilized while practicing Reiki.

Level 2 helps practitioners learn new techniques of channeling energy, such as the method of being able to draw the symbols and send healing energy to others even when they are in the same room.

As for the Level 2 attunement, the intensity is quite high since this is where the student will begin to open the central channel. That's why Reiki masters have recommended to wait for at least 21 days up to three months before trying to jump from the first level to the second one. Once the waiting time is over, the students at Level 2 can undertake the attunement process.

Another thing to take note of the Level 2 attunement is that the Reiki symbols for power, harmony, and distance are given to a student by the Reiki master to indicate that they are finally being passed onto them.

It is not common, but it has been said that some Reiki masters even combine the lessons of Level 1 and 2 together.

Third Degree (Inner Master)

Finally, the third degree or Level 3 of Reiki represents a student's mastery. Known as the Inner Master, the student becomes the teacher at this point. Mostly referred as a Reiki master, this is when they can become the practitioner.

By reaching Level 3, the student will not only learn more methods but also gain the opportunity to attune others. In this way, the newly-appointed master can pass on what they have learned to help others achieve their goals as well.

The Level 3 attunement, commonly referred to as the Master Attunement, will have the practitioner open up energy channels on a much deeper level than what was achieved in Levels 1 and 2. To put it in a simpler way, it is where the session will get more intense than usual. Just like in Level 2, one must wait for a while before undertaking the Level 3 attunement.

With all this being said, it is important to remember that not all of the Reiki masters teach the same way. Even when they are practicing the Usui Reiki method, they may add some moves and guidelines that are not seen in the traditional way. So, make sure to do your research and pick the Reiki master whom you feel will bring you closer to your goals.

How to Ascend Through Reiki Levels

Unlike other alternative healing methods, ascending through the levels or degrees of Reiki healing has a process. First, when you have learned what you need to know from Level 1, you must go through an attunement process with a certified Reiki master who has already achieved the highest level. Second, you will take courses that will help you achieve the succeeding levels. This means you will study the lessons, practice methods, and understand other essential things that will assist you along the journey. You will also learn the distinctive points of the levels and how vital they are when mastering Reiki and integrating the symbols.

Once the time passes after your Level 1 attunement, you can undertake the Level 2 attunement. After that, you will become a Reiki master by the time you achieve Level 3. This is where you will tackle your master attunement task and become recognized as a real practitioner. From there, you can help others who would like to achieve the same thing and give them their attunement as well. You can even put up your own practice and become a practitioner like the other Reiki masters across the globe.

Keep in mind that when you are ascending through the Reiki levels, you need to be patient and observant. You cannot rush through all of them at once. Instead, take your sweet time and let yourself be one with the process. This will also give you a chance to apply what you have learned and practice everything. It will come in handy when you start learning the new healing techniques later.

Remember that your journey doesn't end even when you become a Reiki master. At Level 3, you will see that it has only begun. More opportunities, pathways, and experiences await you now.

Chapter 7: Reiki Healing Hand Positions for a Healthier and Better Life

How Reiki Healing Works: The Theory

When looked at from the most obvious level, it is clear that Reiki treatment has a direct impact on lowering stress levels and releasing tension from the system. Further than this, it also helps a person move towards a better balance in body, mind and spirit. Even more, it can help the body's own natural healing mechanisms to kick in again and begin to function more effectively.

What Exactly Is Reiki Doing?

So, the question is, how does Reiki lower stress and help enable the body to heal? An exact answer to this question remains to be found. However, there have been increasing levels of research covering the effects of Reiki. There is now evidence showing its effect on lowering heart rate, blood pressure, and stress hormones. It has also been shown to improve immune strength. While we have evidence to show the effects

Reiki has, we can only offer broad theories as to what causes these effects and how exactly the healing is occurring.

Reiki affects us on multiple levels and often with immediate results. This suggests that Reiki is a complex process that interacts with many of the body's systems simultaneously. It results in the body shifting from a stressed state, also known as fight-or-flight mode, to one of relaxation, where the body is primed to heal itself–this is referred to as a parasympathetic state. Many scientists suggest that this shift is triggered on a subconscious level in an area referred to as the biofield.

What Is the Biofield?

The biofield refers to an area that surrounds the physical body. Medical science has adopted the term to explain the vibrational energy field that is believed to exist in this space. There is no way of actually studying the biofield as current technology is not yet capable of verifying its existence. Having said this, traditional and indigenous cultures have recognized this biofield of energy for thousands of years, and it has always been believed to be a cornerstone of health and wellbeing. Any disruption to this biofield was seen as a loss in balance and the beginning of an illness. So, just because science has not developed far enough to examine this phenomenon, it does not mean it should be dismissed. The wisdom from indigenous cultures runs much deeper than science, which is a relatively new faculty in terms of human history.

Many healing traditions from indigenous cultures use vibration to restore the necessary balance to the mind and body. We can see evidence of this in practices such as ceremonial drumming, chanting rituals, and humming. There is plenty of science to support the therapeutic benefits of vibration through music and sounds. This has led musicians to purposely construct music that can raise or lower people's energies to the desired level. One song called Weightless was developed by Marconi Union to help relieve stress. The song is said to decrease stress levels by up to 60% once listened to with closed eyes. You can feel the vibrational shift through listening to the song as your body's natural rhythm realigns itself. Some say that Reiki's healing benefits are derived from a similar vibrational mechanism, one which increases the level of coherence in the body and decreases the level of dissonance.

Another theory suggests that a Reiki practitioner's hands hold the power of the energetic vibrations which are transmitted to the recipient. These vibrations are then passed from the practitioner to the client to induce healing. The effect could then cause the client to have a shift in awareness as they recognize the healing power they hold within is the key to their wellbeing, regardless of their current state of health. Reiki could then be seen as helping a person resync back to health, similar to how grandfather clocks in the same room adjust to the rhythm of the main clock or how we, too, become relaxed in the presence of someone who is very peaceful. Reiki can connect the practitioner with a deep, inner peace regardless of how they are feeling at that moment.

Many other therapies aim to restore the biofield's balance. These include yoga, acupuncture, qigong, and shiatsu to name but a few. Reiki is one of the most subtle of these therapies as it uses mainly vibrations rather than physical manipulation or even gentle force. It is also suggested by some that Reiki does not act in the biofield at all but rather another field known as the unified field. Some believe that Reiki is more similar to meditation than other energy therapies.

Reiki Compared to Other Treatments

According to the NCCIH, Reiki is an alternative medicine practice that complements existing practices by using energy that is still to be measured by science. Most energy healing methods presume that humans inhabit a certain type of energy which both runs through us and around us. It is believed that energy therapies such as Healing Touch help to bring equilibrium to these energies.

As mentioned, many Reiki practitioners see Reiki as completely distinct to most energy healing and more akin to meditative practices. Many energy healing methods use specific ways to gain access to a person's biofield to make alterations; Reiki does not try to diagnose problems or purposely alter the energy field. They are more passive in their involvement as the energy finds its path.

Reiki practice by nature is extremely passive. A practitioner's hand does not move for most of the treatment duration. The only time they do is alter placements of the hands. A Reiki practitioner is a neutral party; they do not make an effort to change a person or change their energy field. A Reiki practitioner does not try to harness and use Reiki energy; they simply rest their hands on a person's body. Sometimes, they will rest their hands just above the body, in cases where there is an open wound or burn that needs to be healed.

The energy that arises in a practitioner's hands comes naturally as it responds to the needs of the individual for balance in certain areas. Because of this, every treatment is tailored to meet the specific needs of that person, although the practitioner often uses a similar process for every session.

Reiki is best administered in a complete session; however, it can also be given in a shorter session to tackle certain points of a person's body. In pressing circumstances, even a few minutes of Reiki makes a big difference.

How Reiki Healing Is Done: The Healing Session

Reiki session has no standard or even a set time limit or exact protocol to be adhered to. It is allowed to be performed by anyone who has received the necessary training. This might be someone who is professionally qualified, but it can also be a healthcare provider or a friend or member of your family; it could even be you. There is also no typical setting required for Reiki. Generally, Reiki works best somewhere quiet, but it can be performed anywhere, regardless of what is going on in the vicinity and no matter what is happening to the person receiving it. A few moments of Reiki often brings relaxation to emergencies. It is often administered directly after injuries occur and even during and after surgeries.

Who Should I See?

To give yourself the best experience possible, you must take the time to do some research before choosing a practitioner that you believe you can be comfortable with. You should decide whether you want to receive Reiki from a friend or a professional you do not know. If you have a friend that you feel very comfortable with, it can help improve the bonding experience. However, if you are not naturally comfortable with strangers, you may want to choose a professional for a greater level of experience. Try to meet with your practitioner beforehand to get a feel for the person and to know what to expect from the session.

Look for a practitioner who describes the process to you clearly and details how they plan to structure the session. This will help you know what to expect when going into the session, and it will make you more at ease. Your personal experience of Reiki will be very different from most others, but if you know what to expect before going in, it always helps.

What Is the Setting?

The most beneficial setting is one where it is quiet and where you will not be disturbed. Most professional Reiki practitioners will have a space dedicated to their practice. If they are doing house calls, they will usually have plenty of knowledge of how best to set up an optimal space. Practitioners often play soft music during sessions to promote relaxation through ambient sounds. If you prefer to have no music, however, do not be afraid to let your practitioner know.

The length of sessions can vary widely. For those receiving Reiki in hospitals and nursing homes, sessions tend to only last around twenty minutes. Professional practitioners provide treatments that last up to ninety minutes. Most Reiki treatments are in between the two.

How Do I Sign Up?

Many practitioners will provide clients with intake forms and will conduct a screening interview beforehand to discover the client's health history or if any underlying issues need to be raised. However, because of the nature of Reiki and its origins, many practitioners avoid these types of processes as they are more associated with mainstream medical practices. Reiki is often seen as more informal and less structured than typical medical procedures. Many times, you will need to fill out a consent form.

Next, the entire process will be explained to you and the practitioner will ask if you have any specific needs or requests. It is your job to inform the practitioner if you suffer from any conditions that may affect the session, especially if lying flat on your back or front will be a problem or if there are any places where you are sensitive to touch. In some more formal places, such as hospitals or healthcare environments, a practitioner may have to ask if they are allowed to use their hands on the body.

What Is Involved in a Session?

A full Reiki session requires the recipient to be lying down or upright in a comfortable chair.

Usually, Reiki is performed with soft touches, where the practitioner's hands are placed in multiple locations. These include the head and front and back of a person's belly area. A practitioner should not put their hands in private places, and they should not feel intrusive.

Extra placements on injured parts of the body may be performed as needed, such as on the arm for a surgical scar. The practitioner can also hold their hands just above the affected area if it is sore to the touch, providing the same treatment benefits.

What Is the Experience Like?

The experience of Reiki is very subjective. Sometimes, the changes are very subtle and not initially noticeable to the recipient. However, there seems to be an array of shared experiences many people feel during a Reiki treatment.

Some people quote a feeling of heat emanating from the practitioner's hands, while others note a refreshingly cool feeling coming from their hands. Some also experience a pulsating effect where the practitioner's hands are placed as waves of energy pulsate and flow through the body.

A lot of people comment on how comforting the experience is. One study reported how recipients regularly felt that they were hovering in an altered state of consciousness while, at the same time, being fully aware of their surroundings and drawn deeply within. Others have reported falling into a deep, meditative state, while some find the experience to be quite dramatic. Some find their first Reiki session to be not very eventful, but they often report feeling good afterward. The usual resulting feeling is one of deep relaxation and an instant release of stress.

Reiki is a compounding practice and even those who do not notice much on their first time, usually get deeper and more profound experiences as they continue their sessions. Aside from the immediate after-effects of Reiki treatment, you may also experience other positive changes in the days afterward. These include better digestion, a more centered feeling as opposed to being reactive, and better and deeper sleep.

What Should I Do During the Session?

Once you have chosen a practitioner that you believe you will feel comfortable with and that has adequate skills and knowledge of Reiki, then there is not much you can do during a session other than to relax and to trust in the practitioner.

If you want to try and improve your Reiki experience however, you can try some of these tips:

- Bring some music that you find relaxing to you.

- Go to the bathroom before the session so that you can lie down comfortably without the distraction of feeling the need to go to the toilet.

- If you are very sensitive to being touched, it might help if you ask the practitioner beforehand what areas they plan to touch so that you know exactly what will happen during the session.

- Tell the practitioner of your requirements before the session starts. If you struggle to lay flat or you have difficulty breathing in certain positions, then let them know and they can work on an alternative. Or if you have had surgery recently and are especially sensitive in an area, let them know so they can avoid causing you pain by touching it. Also, if you happen to be pregnant or are suffering from digestive problems, you may not be able to lie on your stomach. Let them know and they can help.

As the session goes on, you should begin to feel more relaxed. If you become uncomfortable, however, be sure to adjust your position. If there is anything else you need to improve your comfort, whether it be a blanket or support for your lower back, make sure to let the practitioner know. This process is designed to help you after all, and the practitioner wants to make sure the experience is as pleasant and comfortable as possible for you.

Do not try to force yourself into relaxation during Reiki. Reiki is a passive experience, and you should naturally be relaxed through the session. Feel free to let your mind wander; listen to the music and your breathing as well as the feelings you experience during the session.

How Does the Session End?

Unlike most other treatments, Reiki does not give a diagnosis, so do not expect one. Practitioners may make some standard recommendations to you such as drink more fluids or to listen to your body.

While most individuals feel refreshed after Reiki, some people note that they feel more tired than usual that evening. This does not mean they reacted badly to the treatment; it is a natural response from the body to be tired after undergoing healing. People often report a rich feeling of calm and clarity after Reiki as well as very good sleep.

What is the Optimum Number of Sessions?

The person you visit might recommend several sessions to you. The traditional number of sessions is four. This tends to give you enough time to evaluate the benefits, if any, you are receiving. You should take the time to discuss how it would be most suitable to arrange the sessions to get the maximum benefits based on your needs and your schedule.

When you are facing a serious illness, most people would suggest a series of four sessions completed in less than one week. They do not necessarily have to be given by the same practitioner.

How Does Reiki Change You: The Effect

Reiki infuses you with love. Reiki can profoundly change your life for the better. People often say that Reiki opens you up to the power of the universe's unconditional love. They feel a humbling sense of connection to everyone and everything around us. This power helps eliminate the fear of failure, rejection, and pain. It can even help eliminate the fear of success, which holds many people back without them knowing it. It also helps to eliminate the restrictions and limitations we have unnecessarily attached to ourselves about what we believe we can and cannot do. Reiki can conquer your fears and limitations. It helps us see the love we have for ourselves and others around us. It reminds us of our connection to all things in the universe.

Reiki chooses you. It is said that Reiki chooses you. Nobody consciously decides to become a Reiki healer; rather, they are drawn to it by a higher power. Being called to Reiki can be overwhelming at first, but it is a path that leads to contentment and peace in what you do. Many teachers talk about how most Reiki students start by saying they are not sure exactly how they got here, but it seems to be how a journey in Reiki starts for most people.

Before the attunement day. The pre-attunement cleansing and healing process can have a big impact on a student's life. Many who have gone through it recommend that students keep a journal for at least a month leading up to the day they are to be attuned. A lot of things that occur may seem insignificant at the time, but they are, in fact, very important. It is only in the weeks after that their value and importance will be clear to see. Looking back at yourself before attunement, you will be able to better understand the difference in how you used to think. Once you make Reiki a part of your regular habit, your views on things change. You have unleashed a talent that was there before but lay undiscovered. Now, you will be able to see life through an entirely new lens.

Becoming free. Reiki can open many doors for people on many levels. This includes emotionally, psychologically, and spiritually. You will develop a skill to notice small inconveniences, and you will not give them the power to disturb your feelings. You will have an ability to see through the many insignificant happenings of the everyday grind that bothers most people. You will be able to free yourself from the small problems that we often build up in front of ourselves to hold us back from living to our full and true capability. Once we begin on the path of Reiki, we experience freedom.

Reiki's blessings. Reiki has a whole host of blessings that continue to evolve. The most obvious of these is the new perspective we gain on our purpose through a spiritual reawakening. We gain an increased clarity of thought and action that enables us to naturally heal and be healed. The real blessing of Reiki is the knowledge we gain about our natural healing abilities and how to use them. Over time, we gain more experience and develop further wisdom about our life purpose as we go along our spiritual path. Reiki is a tool that enables us to live in this way.

Recognizing the connection to the greatness of spirit. Reiki improves your everyday experience for the better. You start feeling more free as you experience the infinite power of the all-knowing. This spirit is what brings life and love to all things.

Chapter 8: Power of Positive Thoughts

The phrase positive thinking sounds wonderful on the surface. Most people would rather have positive thoughts than negative ones. This phrase is a fluffy one that is usually dismissed in the real world. It doesn't carry the same weight as a phrase like hard working or work ethic. These views are changing.

Research and people are telling us that positive thinking isn't just about being happy, or pasting a smile on your face to everyone to see. Positive thoughts add real value to your everyday life and can help build skills that will last longer than a pasted-on smile.

A positive psychology researcher from the University of North Carolina, Barbara Fredrickson has helped to prove the power of positive thoughts on everyday life. Let's look at what she found and what it means for you.

Let's take a look at what negative thoughts can do to your brain. Imagine this.

Pretend you are walking in the woods. A tiger suddenly appears before you on the path. When you see the tiger, your brain automatically creates a negative emotion. For this example, it is fear.

Researchers have known for a long time that negative responses can cause you to act a certain way. Such as if a tiger crosses your path, you are going to run. Nothing else matters in that moment. Your attention is on the tiger, the fear, and how you plan on getting away.

This means that a negative emotion will narrow the focus of your mind and thoughts. At this moment, you could choose to grab a stick, climb a tree, or pick up a leaf. Your brain ignores these options because they aren't relevant when you have a tiger standing in front of you.

This is a wonderful thing to have if you need to save yourself, but in today's world, you don't have to fear walking up on a tiger in the woods. The bad news is, the brain still has a programmed response to negative emotion, and it will shut out the rest of the world and will limit what you see.

One other example is if you are fighting with someone. The anger and emotions you feel might completely consume you, and you won't be able to think about anything else. If you are stressing out about everything you need to get done today, you might find it hard to focus on what you need to do or how to get started because the length of your list has you paralyzed. You might feel bad because you haven't been eating right or exercising. All you can think about is your willpower and thinking that you are lazy. This is causing you to not have any motivation.

With all of these examples, your brain shuts off to the outside world and just focuses on the emotions of stress, anger, and fear, just like with the tiger. The only thing negative emotions do is prevents your brain from seeing other options that might be around you. This is a survival instinct.

So, what do positive thoughts do to the brain?

Fredrickson created an experiment to see if positive emotions impacted the brain. In this experiment, she divided her subjects into five separate groups and showed them different movie clips.

Two groups were shown clips that created positive emotions. One group was shown things that caused tremendous joy. The other group was shown things that created contentment.

The third group was the control group, and they were shown things that caused no significant emotional change.

The last two groups were shown clips that caused negative emotions. One of the last groups saw images that created fear; the other was shown things to cause anger.

Once they had seen the images, all participants were asked to picture themselves in a place that would cause the same emotions to come up and write down what they would do. They were given a sheet of paper that had 20 fill-ins the blank lines that started with "I would like to…"

The participants that were shown images that caused fear and anger were not able to write down as many responses. The participants that were shown images that caused contentment and joy could write down a lot more actions than even the control group.

This means if you feel positive emotions like love, joy, or contentment, you will see more things that you could do in life. The findings showed that positive emotions could broaden your sense of possibilities and open your mind.

More interesting discoveries came later.

Benefits from positive emotions don't end when the emotion ends. You receive the most benefits from these emotions with an ability to build greater skills that you could use later in life.

Children that run outside, swing in tree branches, and play with friends are developing physical, social, and creative skills by moving athletically, playing and communicating with others, and learning how to explore the world. This happens because the emotions of joy and play are prompting the child to build these skills that will be useful to them later in life.

These skills will last them longer than the actual emotions that initiated the learning. Negative emotions have a different effect since building skills for the future are irrelevant to the brain in a moment when you are faced with immediate danger or a threat.

These thoughts and emotions can greatly impact your life. It is important that you learn more about positive thinking.

Don't misunderstand what is meant by positive thinking. This doesn't mean that you turn a blind eye to the bad things in life. Positive thinking means that you approach unpleasant moments positively and productively. You must believe that only the best will happen.

Thinking positively starts with self-talk. If you don't know what this is, it is the stream of unspoken communication that goes through your mind. These thoughts can be negative or positive. Self-talk can come from reason or logic. It can arise from misconceptions because the lack of information that you have about something.

If your self-talk is mostly negative, then your outlook is going to be pessimistic. If your self-talk is positive, then you will be more optimistic.

Researchers continue to explore all the effects that optimism and positive thinking has on health. Here are some of the benefits:

- Better coping skill when facing stress or hardships.

- Improved cardiovascular health and reduced risk of dying from heart disease.

- Improved physical and psychological well-being.

- More resistance to getting a cold.

- Lower stress levels.

- Lower depression levels.

- A longer life.

Negative self-talk comes in one of these forms:

Polarizing

You see things as either only good or only bad. There is no middle ground. You feel like you have to be perfect or you are a failure.

Catastrophizing

Your thoughts will go automatically to the worst-case scenario. Your regular coffee shop gets your order wrong, and you think that the rest of your day will be horrible.

Personalizing

If something goes wrong, or something bad happens, you automatically blame yourself. Here's an example, your friend's night out gets canceled. You automatically think it is because no one wants to be around you, so everyone canceled.

Filtering

You increase the negative parts of a situation and ignore the positive ones. For example, you had a great day at work. You got all your work done faster than normal, and your boss compliments you on the quality of work and how fast you got it done. That evening, you can only think about doing more tasks the next day and totally forget the compliments you received from your boss.

No need to fret, it is easy to change your negative thoughts with positive ones. It will take some time and effort. It is just like creating a new habit. Here are a few ways you can get started:

- Find areas that need to be changed.

If you want to become more optimistic and practice positive thinking, find the places in your life where you are always negative. This might be your commute to work, a relationship, or basically anything. Begin by focusing on just one area.

- Check yourself.

Every now and then check in with yourself during the day and see what you are thinking about. If you see that your thoughts are negative, figure out a way you can turn them positive.

- Learn to love humor.

Give yourself permission to laugh and smile, especially if you are going through a hard time. Find humor in everything that happens throughout the day. If you can learn to laugh at life, you will feel less stressed.

- Start a healthy lifestyle

Start exercising about 30 minutes a few days a week. If you don't have the time to do 30 minutes at one time, break it up into three ten-minutes sets. Exercise creates a positive effect on your mood and can help you reduce stress. Eating a healthy diet can help fuel your body and mind.

- Surround yourself with positive things.

Be sure the people you spend time with will add positive feelings to your life. They need to be supportive and positive. They need to provide you with helpful feedback and advice. If you surround yourself with negative people, it will increase your stress and negativity.

- Practice positive self-talk

Try to follow this rule: Never say things that you wouldn't say to a friend. You need to be encouraging and gentle. If negative thoughts do enter your mind, look at them rationally and say a positive affirmation. Think of things that you are thankful for.

Chapter 9: Reiki and Meditation

Meditation is a common practice in Reiki. Many holistic healers and practitioners do include meditation of some kind in their lives. Whether they are yoga instructors, massage therapists, Reiki practitioners, or individuals that are committed to a full body, mind, and spirit wellness will use meditation regularly.

There are two basic forms of meditation. The first is to completely clear your mind of all thoughts. The second type of meditation is to focus on a specific question, concern, or situation.

With Reiki meditation, the focus is on Reiki energy rather than any other subject. During a Reiki meditation, you focus on the universal energy as it is within you, around you, and within everything around you. You want to feel connected to that energy to create a feeling of tranquility, connection, and peace.

Your body will feel revitalized and full of life energy. It is a very rejuvenating type of meditation.

When you meditate, it is recommended that you find a quiet place where you won't be disturbed. You'll want to set a relaxing atmosphere. Set the lights low, light some candles, maybe burn some incense or diffuse herbal oils. If music helps you relax, play a soothing soundtrack.

You can sit or lie down for meditation, but if you are prone to falling asleep, sitting up may be the best idea. While it isn't bad to fall asleep during meditation, the goal is to keep a certain focus and connection with the Reiki energy which won't be as strong if you fall asleep.

To start relaxing your mind, breathe in through your nose to the count of four and then breathe out through your mouth to the count of eight.

After a few of these deep breaths, you'll want to start focusing on Reiki energy. Start with the energy within yourself, and as you connect to it, feel it expand outward into the universe and into the space and objects around you. You should feel the energy moving through you and around you.

Keep your focus on that energy for as long as you want to, or as long as you feel called to. If you want to meditate for a certain amount of time, set some kind of timer with a gentle call back sound like a soft bell or gong to let you when you should end the meditation.

Meditation can take practice. If you are unfamiliar with meditation or new to meditation, you might have to work your way up to longer meditation times. Starting with just five minutes is fairly standard.

In the beginning, it is easy to get distracted by thoughts and sounds in the room around you, like the heat coming on, the sound of a branch on the window, or thoughts of your day. Over time, with practice, these distractions won't be as prominent.

However, there are some techniques to help you stay in that meditative mindset. One method to try is when you begin to meditate, set the tip of your tongue to the top of your mouth. If your mind starts to wander, your tongue will fall from the roof of your mouth. Any time you notice this, bring your tongue back to the roof of your mouth and refocus on your meditation.

The tongue trick is somewhat similar to the Gassho finger technique in which you press your middle fingers together if you begin to experience thoughts that pull you away from your meditation. Starting a meditation with the Gassho technique can also help your mind focus when you move into a Reiki meditation.

There is a somewhat standard 21-day Reiki meditation program that can help you learn more about Reiki and also help you develop your meditation skills. It is broken down into different segments to cover the 21 days. These 21 days are also symbolic of the time that Dr. Usui spent on top of a mountain in study to reach enlightenment.

Chapter 10: Reiki and Body Energy

Everything is about energy, which means that healing also ultimately involves energy. In Reiki, energy helps promote healing through enhancing the flow of energy and correcting any disturbances that occur in the "human energy field," also called the aura. This aura permeates the body and surrounds it. When the body experiences the flow of energy, the body will have the capacity to heal by itself.

Energy healing works on the basis that your body is made up of various patterns of energy. When you work directly with body energy, you will influence the mental, physical, and emotional level. Using energy healing in Reiki is seen to be holistic in nature.

This is why it is vital that when your body or mind experiences disturbances, everyone wants to address these levels. However, energy healing doesn't work on its own; rather, it supports other healing methods that we use in daily life. Reiki healing focuses on the energy of which your body, mind, and emotions are made up of.

At the center of the human field are seven primary chakras that are supported by thousands of other smaller meridians and chakras. The seven chakras are placed vertically along your spinal column, and it begins on the pelvic floor. The first one is the Root chakra that is at the level of the pelvic bone, and the one at the top is the crown chakra. Each of the chakras works as its own transmitter as well as the recipient of the energy. When the chakra receives the energy, it will direct it to corresponding organs as well as the endocrine system within the body.

The Energetic Bodies

In addition to the chakra, the human body uses the human energy field to make it work perfectly. The energy field is made up of smaller energetic bodies, which include the mental, spiritual, etheric, emotional, and physical bodies. All these allow you to relate with and experience the environment in different aspects.

When all the chakras and energy bodies are in harmony and are working well together, you will be full of vitality and have a sense of wellness. On the other hand, when the energy centers are not balanced, you will become sluggish, and you will experience confusion, fatigue, and illness at all times. You need to work with a healing practice that can identify the problem areas. He will do so to release the blockages then create a positive flow of energy in the body so that he can make you heal. Healing can happen immediately, or it can take time.

The 5 Layers of the Human Energy Field

Physical Energy

This is the layer that we look at to be the physical part of ourselves. Although we look at the body as a package that consists of the skin, flesh, bones, and organs, they also have energy, similar to the other layers of the body that you can't see, or you cannot sense such as the mind.

Etheric

This word is derived from the word "ether," – which is a layer that sits from one quarter to one half of an inch but not any more than an inch, from the location of the physical body. The practitioners that have sensed this body describe it as a feeling that is gray in color. It is like a spider web, and it can stretch, and it is usually seen as the blueprint of the physical layer.

Emotional Energy

This is the third layer from the outside. It is at the center of all the five layers that we have looked at. The emotional layer is the layer where fears and feelings reside. It can be very volatile when we have emotions. It comes into play whether you are experiencing both low and high emotions.

Mental Energy

This is the layer where our ideas and other emotions spring from. It also forms the store from which the belief system gets stored. This is the space where our thoughts are stored then sorted out, and it is where people store their personal truths or any perceptions that are based on experiences.

Spiritual Energy

This is the final layer, where higher awareness and consciousness is stored. It is the layer where our past lives are tied as well as the universal consciousness that is common to all people.

Why Should You Be Concerned About Energy Field?

You need to be aware that the personal energy field has a huge impact on the general sense of wellbeing. People are usually aware of how important personal hygiene is. You need to know that the physical body gets dirty when you use it, and it can pick up viruses and bacteria that can lead to disease. If you stop looking after your body, your physical health, as well as a sense of wellbeing, will also suffer.

Have you ever felt that your state of mind feels "dirty" when your body is dirty as well? This is because everything that you do is connected to the energy, which also means that every part of your life comes with an energy component. Visible dirt is just a part of the bigger problem. Any part of your body is made up of many energy frequencies, most which cannot be seen with the naked eye. However, you need to know that the unseen energy frequencies will affect the energy field as well.

The major problem that we face is that we have grown up in a society that doesn't acknowledge the unseen energies and how they are important to our lives. In school, we are only taught about the energies that we can see, and how they affect our lives, we aren't taught about what we cannot see.

For you to understand how it all works, you need to look at all the five layers of the human energy fields. It is a fact that for you to have total body hygiene, you ought to keep all the five layers of body energy clean. When you know the different fields, you will be able to know that the conditions in your body that you think is caused by physical causes might be due to energy imbalance. You don't need to limit yourself at a single part of the body; rather, you need to look at the different layers before you make any conclusion. If you wish to handle the proper healing of the body, you need to do so by working at all the layers of the body.

Chapter 11: Reiki for Yourself and Others

Once you are familiar with Reiki healing and have sufficient practice on healing yourself, you can move on and try healing others. Anyone who begins Reiki healing is eager to help others with their newfound skill. In this chapter, you will learn more about how you can give Reiki to other people. You can go your own way when you master all the techniques. You can then trust your instinct and skills to treat someone properly with Reiki.

Remember to put yourself first. This is not the same as being selfish and is all about self-care. No one is responsible for caring for you but you. Before a healer heals others, they must heal themselves. Keep this in mind. You need to learn how to relax and be good to yourself. Make time in your schedule to practice Reiki on yourself every day; the results will make you eager to continue doing so. The level 1 Reiki class in Reiki training will teach you all about practicing Reiki on yourself. Follow the class structure and make sure you regularly practice Reiki healing on yourself.

As you keep practicing, you will discover the benefits of conducting Reiki on yourself. It will make you familiar with Reiki healing. Regular Reiki will help to maintain high levels of health in your body and good mental health as well. You will be more open and be a better Reiki channel. You will also be setting your outlook to one that is more open to receiving intuition. Try putting aside some time every morning to practice Reiki before you do anything else. It can be done before you even get out of bed. Also do this before you go to sleep every night. Use all the techniques that have been mentioned. Use meditation as an important tool. Use intention to keep the energy flowing, and hone your intuition to know how you should be moving your hands. Remember that integrity is an important aspect.

When you move on to healing others, there are a lot of things to keep in mind. The recipient is placing their trust and faith in you; honor their trust and expectation. Do not practice Reiki until you are sure of your skills. Make people as comfortable as possible during the session. If the patient says that they don't want to lie down, give them a place to sit comfortably. Reiki can still be conducted in this position. Take time to communicate and find out what the recipient is expecting from this Reiki session. Ask them about any pains and troubles they have been facing as well. Ask them to wear some comfortable clothing so that they can relax completely during the session.

You can begin giving hands-on healing to the person when they are properly relaxed and comfortable. Use the various Reiki hand positions to heal them with Reiki. Begin the session by practicing Reiki over the crown chakra. This will help in the energy flow and allow them to enter a deeply relaxing state. Then start treating the chakras in the front. The next stage is to balance out the energy in the body. You can use spiraling as a tool for this. Ask the person to turn over and then begin healing the chakras at the back of the body. Repeat the balancing exercise. Then continue with any specific healing according to whatever illness or pains the recipient has informed you of.

You can also use distant healing on other people. This can only be done by a Reiki practitioner who has been attuned to level 3 Reiki or the Master level. Distant healing can be carried out by using different techniques like using photographs, surrogates, imagination, intention slips, etc.

Hand Positions in Reiki

Before you begin healing others, get sufficient practice in using your hands for healing yourself. This is one of the first steps to start with. The hand positions will be nearly the same even when you practice Reiki on someone else.

You will now learn about the hand positions that are derived from the Reiki practiced by Hawayo Takata and her students. There are other hand positions taught by Mikao Usui or Hayashi that you can explore as well. The hand positions will usually be similar to the ones that are commonly used in western Reiki practices. Ultimately, you should begin with any hand positions so that you can use your intuition as a guide. The spirit will guide you in moving your hands where they are really needed.

- Follow these guidelines before you delve into hand positions.

- The Reiki recipient should be made comfortable. Let them lie on their back on a good massage table.

- As the Reiki giver, you should be standing or sitting. Choose a position that is comfortable and will allow you to perform Reiki well.

- There should be enough space around the table for you to walk around it.

- Try keeping your fingers together as you carry out all the Reiki positions.

- When you move from one position to another, do it gently.

- When you work on any organs or chakras, study about them to learn more.

- Keep all the ethical considerations in mind when you practice Reiki on another person.

Hand Positions for Each Region in the Body

The Head

Start at the top or the head. This is the position that you should begin with if the patient suffers from headaches, colds and allergies, toothaches, earaches, etc. It is also where you should concentrate if the person suffers from a lot of stress. It will help to establish balance throughout the body. The hand positions on the head are more important than any other.

At the eyes and face, keep your hands over the closed eyes of the recipient. Keep your hands on both sides of the nose. Rest your fingers on the cheekbone. Let your thumbs rest together over the third eye. You can also use a tissue to protect the eyes.

At the top of the head, keep your hands lying over this region. Both your wrists should be touching, and the fingers of each hand should be pointing downward towards the corresponding ears. Try to hover over the crown region and keep your hands away from their hair if you want. Keep your hands here for a while to ensure that the crown chakra is open.

At the temples, keep your hands rested on either side of the forehead. Your hands should be between their hairline and eyebrows with the fingers resting lightly on the cheekbones. This hand position will help to balance the brain and increase the spiritual connectivity.

At the ears, keep your hands over each ear. It will help to calm the mind and treat an illness related to the ears.

Behind their head, you should move your hands under the head. Roll the person's head to the opposite side as you place your hands there one by one. Your fingers should just be touching at the top of their neck while you are holding the medulla oblongata region.

Front of the Body

Now let us move down to the front of the body. This will include the throat and the neck, which act as a transition point between your head and upper body.

At the throat, use your hands to gently cup the bottom of their throat while letting the tips of your fingers touch. Don't touch the throat but keep your hands around it. This hand position will help you in healing the thyroid and parathyroid issues with Reiki. It can be used for treating the larynx, vocal cords, and lymph nodes as well. Remember that some patients might not be comfortable with your hands around their throat so keep your hands a little further away to accommodate them.

At the collarbone, keep your hands rested on either side of the neck; your fingers should be pointing towards the center of the chest. You can give Reiki to the thymus region with this hand position. It plays an important role in immunity.

At the back of the neck or in front of the heart, there is a different position. Keep your left hand under the neck, and the right hand should be placed over the top of the heart. This hand position heals the heart and throat chakra at the same time.

At the heart, keep your hands in a "T" position. One hand has to be placed horizontally over the patient's breast while the other has to be in between the breasts. This position will help to heal the heart chakra. Any issues with the circulatory system, lungs, and thymus gland will require this hand position. You will be able to increase the flow of loving energy with Reiki with it.

At the upper abdominal region, keep your hands straight under the chest area. Use this hand position while performing Reiki on the spleen or any digestive organs. It will also treat the solar plexus chakra.

At the middle abdomen, keep your hands a little further down compared to the previous position under the chest. One hand should be above the navel while the other should be below it. Illness of the pancreas, intestines, and gallbladder will require this hand position.

At the sacral and lower abdominal region, keep your hands on the lower abdomen. Each hand should be placed in front of the other. Make sure your hands are away from the genital region. The sacral chakra is healed with this hand position. You can also use it while healing the pelvic region, bladder, and any reproductive issues.

Back of the Body

The next hand positions are for the back of the body. The recipient has to turn over for this. If they are in a deep state of rest, give them some time and calmly ask them to change positions. This position will give you easier access to some chakras in the body and helps treat any back issues.

At the upper shoulders, keep your hands under their neck and on top of each shoulder. It will help to relieve tension in this region and is also helpful to treat the throat chakra.

At the shoulder blades, move your hands a few inches down and keep them rested on top of the shoulder blades. Use this position while healing the heart chakra or any issues with lungs or heart in the recipient.

At the waist area, place both your hands. You can use it while treating the solar plexus chakra, kidneys, and adrenal gland.

At the lower back region, keep your hands rested on the hollow of their back, above the buttock region. Use this position for releasing tension in the lower back and for treating the sacral chakra.

Legs and Feet

Lastly, you have the positions for the legs and feet. Originally, there were no standard positions for this region. You can continue with treating these areas while the person is still lying on their front and their back faces you. You can either sit near their feet or choose to stand, depending on which position is comfortable for you.

At the knees, use your hands to hold them on either side. You can cup the knee from both sides with your hands and treat patients with any knee pain or injury.

While treating the ankles, keep each hand on each ankle. This hand position helps balance the energy of both the legs.

For the soles of the feet, firmly place each hand on the back of each foot. This hand position will have a grounding effect and helps to bring balance to the body.

Using Hand Positions for Physical Healing

Eyes

You can use Reiki to treat any ailments related to the eye like cataracts or glaucoma. Take a paper napkin and cover the eyes with it. Use your fingers to move over the eyes and then to the side of the head. Then move your fingers to the back of the head. For some people, it may take just a few sessions to treat their condition, but others might require months. It is advisable to carry this out for at least fifteen minutes every day to see results.

Nose

Here I will tell you how you can practice Reiki over the region of the nose. Take a paper napkin and cover the nose with it without blocking the nostrils. Use your hands to move over the nose and then the cheekbones from where you move to the forehead, and lastly, the top of the head.

Ears

Take your hands and place them over the ears. Put a finger in each ear. Then move the patient to the side and place your hand behind their ear. Do this on the other ear as well after turning them to the other side. The solar plexus, as well as the throat region, should be healed when addressing ailments with the ears.

When the session is over, the ears should be cleaned out, and eyes washed.

Voicebox

You can also use Reiki to heal the voice box and build up the voice. At the place where the throat joins the shoulder, place your hand, and practice healing all over the throat.

Teeth and Gums

Place your hand over both the jaws and move them to cover all the teeth. The gums will also get tightened as the healing starts working. This also addresses any concerns in the mouth or tongue.

Goiter

The solar plexus and the kidney need to be healed. Use your hands for healing at the location of the goiter near the root of the neck. Digestion needs to be improved, and the heart also has to be treated.

Warts and Polyps

Place your hands over warts or polyps as you use Reiki. With time, they will detach and fall off right from the roots. When polyps are physically cut off, the roots remain and they recur. Reiki healing helps to complete uprooting and removal.

Migraines

Wrong nutrition is usually the reason for headaches from migraine. This is why you need to heal the kidneys and stomach for this. Also focus on the top, back, and sides of the head along with the throat.

Balding and Hair Loss

Proper diet is essential to treat this along with Reiki.

Asthma

Find the place at the root of the throat where the throat joins the shoulders, and place your hands there. Then move to the underside of the jaws to the cheeks and nose. For a female, you should address healing of the ovaries and for a male, the prostate.

By now you are familiar with hand positions that are used while performing Reiki on every region of the recipient's body. There are some additional Reiki positions that you can learn as well. Remember to respect the boundaries of the recipient. If they are uncomfortable with any position, switch instantly. Don't try to force them at any point. On sensitive regions like the genitals or breasts, keep the hands hovering above the region and try avoiding any direct contact. Reiki can always be conducted without touching the body, so respect all ethical boundaries.

Chapter 12: Affirmations

An affirmation is a positive sentence that will affect your conscious and subconscious mind. Repeating an affirmation has the power of helping it manifest. If you visualize and repeat your affirmation continuously, it will help in the manifestation of your desires much faster. Using affirmations with Reiki will make the result more profound.

Positivity plays a very important role in your life. People probably tell you to stay positive all the time while assuring you that everything will be fine. There is more to this than just words. Positive thoughts and energy can be very powerful. If you focus on the bad things and negative thoughts in your life, this will result in the manifestation of those.

Thinking and acting positively will therefore help in the manifestation of positive results in your life. I'm not saying that a miracle will happen and you will get an expensive car just by saying you will get it the next day; however, if that car is what you want, use it in your affirmation sentence. When you practice Reiki and repeat this affirmation over time, it will help you get that car. You may be wondering how this is possible. Well, when you focus on that car or just anything else, you know what you want.

Reiki and meditation will help to change your mindset and life to a much more positive one. This will make it possible to be determined and work singularly until you achieve your goal of buying that car. This is how the manifestation will work in your favor. When you keep lamenting your bad luck or anything negative, your energy and thoughts are focused on those. This drains you of the positive energy required to live your life more productively. Can you understand a little now?

Negative thoughts can arise at any moment, and they may be very overwhelming at times; however, with the help of Reiki, you can exercise control over these thoughts and turn them into more positive ones. Your negative thoughts should never overpower the positivity in you. For this, you need to maintain balance in your chakras, lead a healthy lifestyle, and practice Reiki regularly.

Healing with Affirmations

Affirmations are an easy and simple tool for healing. There is no complicated formula, symbol, or technique involved. This is why it is one of the easiest tools to use in your daily life, but it has a profound impact.

One of the ways to heal with affirmations is to chant. Chanting is a practice that is used all over the world and in various religions. Just repeating certain words with complete faith has a way of harnessing power into them. This is why you should try repeating your affirmation like a chant whenever you get a chance.

Use the affirmation chant to charge a bottle of water or some crystal that you can carry with you all day. You can also write the affirmation on some paper and place a glass of water over it. This water can be consumed or sprayed around your space when it is charged with the affirmation.

Another method involves using Reiki more proactively. Write your affirmation on a paper and then practice Reiki over it with your palms. You can either hold the affirmation paper or hover over it with your hands. You can also do this by keeping a bottle of water on the table. Now use your palms to hover over this bottle. Invoke Reiki and the associated symbols as you chant the affirmation. Try visualizing the outcome of your affirmation while you move your hands over the water. This also helps to charge that bottle of water with positive energy, and you can continue consuming it throughout the day.

Meditating on an affirmation is a healthy and effective practice. Take time out every day to meditate over your desired goal. Sit in a peaceful place and take some calming breaths. Close your eyes and begin chanting the affirmation. Meditate on the outcome that you desire. Visualize it happening. This can be a powerful tool and will strengthen your belief in the possibility of the affirmation manifesting.

Using crystals is another great alternative to try. Find the appropriate crystal for your purpose and cleanse it before you use it. Crystals absorb energy from each person they come in contact with, and you need to make sure the crystal you use is cleansed for your purpose. Now hold the crystal in your palms and use Reiki to charge it. Focus and use your complete concentration to repeat your affirmation as you hold the crystal. Direct the affirmation into the crystal and manifest the energy from your third-eye chakra. Visualize a white light coming from your chakra and beaming into the crystal. Then imagine the outcome of your affirmation happening. Use this charged crystal and keep it in a sacred space. You can also choose to carry it with you at all times.

All of the ways given above are just some of the options available to you. You can heal with affirmations in many ways. The affirmation that you create in the first place should be a powerful and meaningful sentence. This does not mean it has to be something complex and long; in fact, it should be a short and clear sentence. Think well about what you want to manifest and then use it as an affirmation.

Chapter 13: Meditations to Help You Align with Reiki

The following meditations are guided to help you answer your own energy healing needs. Whether you have been attuned to Reiki or not, you can begin to use the principles, pillars, and other tools of Reiki to align better with channeling the energy all around you for healing purposes. You can give yourself all of the healing efforts that you need with these simple instructions and mediations.

For all of these meditation experiences, you will need to find a quiet and comfortable space to help you feel connected to your energy and provide an undisturbed atmosphere of relaxation and relief. You can put on some soothing music and light some incense and candles to create the healing energy all around you.

For some, sitting in a chair or in a cross-legged pose on the floor will be comfortable, while others may want to lie down on a floor mat or other comfortable furniture. Choose the space that allows you to feel the most focused and relaxed.

These three guided meditations are meant to be used on a regular basis to help you treat your own healing needs. Using them only once or twice won't have a lasting benefit and you will need to use them regularly if you are looking for results.

Meditation to Heal the Auric Field

This meditation is designed to help you focus on the auras of the energetic body. You can use it with your own practices or simply follow these guidelines.

In a comfortable position, begin with a Mu-Shin gassho.

Recite the 5 Principles of Reiki in your mind.

Just for today, I will not worry.

Just for today, I will not be angry.

Just for today, I will do my work honestly.

Just for today, I will give thanks for my many blessings.

Just for today, I will be kind to every living thing.

Take many deep breaths, in and out, for a few moments and center yourself.

Close your eyes and continue your breaths.

Through your third eye, look at your auric field and begin to see its color and light. Try not to decide what it should look like; only try to see what it is showing you.

As you start to gain focus on your auric field, allow yourself to discover if there is anything visible that looks unwanted, unnecessary, unhealthy, or destructive to your energy. It could be dark spots, shadowy blocks, people, places, or things. Keep in mind and remember that Reiki allows you to see through your subconscious consciously and so you will want to just let whatever comes up to exist.

When you have identified a mysterious element or several, begin to focus on the palms of your hands and the crown of your head. See light energy coming through the top of your head and traveling through your whole body.

Let the light coming through your crown begin to beam out of the palms of your hands. When you see that light coming through your palms, begin to direct your hands to the areas of your auric field that have any spots that need healing.

Gently place your healing hands over the spot you recognize in your auric field. Send Reiki energy into the spot and stay here until you feel ready to move to the next spot.

Continue to do this until all of your "aura spots" have been removed or cleared.

Reexamine your auric field and make sure that you have released any dark spots or debris (again it could appear as something not described here).

With everything removed, let your hands relax next to you on the floor if you are lying down, or on your lap if you are seated.

Now see the light beaming through your crown as a golden light. See it sparkle and shimmer as it fills your whole body.

Let this golden light seep out of your skin and envelop all of your auric fields, out to the causal layer.

Spend several breaths allowing this golden light to fill your entire energetic space.

When you are ready, present a Mu-shin gassho, give thanks to the Reiki for guiding you, and release yourself from the meditation.

Drink a glass of clean water and rest for several minutes reflecting on your experience.

Use this meditation several days a week to kick start your self-healing experience.

Meditation to Heal the Karmic Past

This meditation can be helpful when you are needing to heal deeper emotional wounds and family patterns that keep you locked in unhealthy cycles and habits. You can use this meditation as often as you need to, and it is recommended daily for at least two weeks to help you resolve deeper emotional issues in your life.

1. Begin your meditation in a lying down position. Use whatever pillows or bolsters you need to support your low back and hips.

2. Bring your attention to your breathing and offer thanks to your healing with the Reiki principles with a simple gassho.

3. Ask for Reiki and Universal life-force energy to guide you on your healing path.

4. Ask for guidance and assistance from your spirit guides and any other Masters of healing in the Universe.

5. Close your eyes and release any tension in your body as you inhale and exhale. Spend a few minutes with this.

6. As you become more relaxed, use your third eye to feel that Reiki energy beaming through your crown and filling your whole body. Let it come to the palms of your hands and the soles of your feet, grounding you and preparing you to heal the past.

7. Either place your palms on your hips, on either side of your root chakra or set them at the very tops of your thighs, as close to your root chakra as you can get (your root chakra is at the base of your spine).

8. See the Reiki energy beaming through the layer of your skin, tissue, muscle, and bone, to your red root chakra energy. Spend time visualizing this healing energy connecting to your root.

9. Allow anything to come up that needs to. You may see flashes of light, images of someone's face, a past memory. You may feel a lot of emotions and may be compelled to cry or feel upset. Try not to avoid the feelings or sensations and just let them rise.

10. As you begin to notice what issues are coming up, see the Reiki energy beaming from your palms connecting to those ideas or visuals. Allow the light energy to dissolve the issue from the past, or the karmic wounds that are lifting up out of your root chakra.

11. Allow plenty of time to experience this meditative part. You may see family in your third eye that you knew as a child or an experience you had. You may feel emotions

that are not attached to a specific image. However it manifests, let the Reiki energy beam light and love through the palms of the hands and into the root chakra.

12. When you feel like there is nothing else coming up for resolve, allow your hands to relax at your sides and breathe for several moments.

13. If your hands feel guided to another chakra after releasing energy from the root, allow your hands to travel to that area and perform the same actions as you did with the root chakra. Let the Reiki field show you what to heal and continue until you are guided to stop.

14. Return to your relaxed position and take several breaths.

15. When you are ready, release the meditation and give gratitude to Reiki with a gassho.

This can be an intense purging and cleansing experience. Be gentle with yourself and your energy afterward and enjoy some simple pleasures, like a walk, or some soothing music with a cup of tea.

Meditation to Awaken the Channels of Light

The last meditation will offer you a special way to ignite the whole chakra system. This is very beneficial for a spiritual awakening practice and also for balancing your entire system for general health and happiness.

Chapter 14: Frequently Asked Questions About Reiki

There are several questions that are commonly asked about Reiki. In this chapter, these questions will be answered to help individuals get a clear and accurate knowledge about the Reiki system.

Where does the Reiki energy originate?

Reiki energy is usually perceived as a subtle energy, which is different from other physical energy, such as chemical energy or electricity. Reiki energy originates from the Higher Power. The Higher Power is found on a dimension, which is higher than the physical world that people have come to know.

When the Reiki energy is perceived in a precognitive manner, it may seem to come down from up above, entering the top of a Reiki practitioner's head. Then, it may appear to flow through the practitioner's body and coming out of the hands. On the other hand, the real source of the Reiki energy is within oneself. The energy comes from a transcendental part of oneself, which is linked to an inexhaustible healing energy supply.

Is the Reiki system a type of religion?

While Reiki is fundamentally spiritual, it is not considered a religion. For one, the Reiki system does not demand practitioners to change their spiritual or religious beliefs. Practitioners have the freedom to preserve what they believe in and make decisions based on the nature of their religious beliefs and practices.

How is a Reiki treatment administered?

In a basic treatment, the Reiki energy flows from a practitioner's hands going to the client. More often than not, the client is lying on a massage table; however, Reiki treatments can also be administered even if the client prefers to stand or sit.

During the treatment, the client is fully clothed. The practitioner directs his or her hands on the client's body, making use of various hand positions. The practitioner usually places his or her hands around the head, stomach, shoulders, and feet of the client. The practitioner can also use more specific positions depending on the needs of the client.

Each position is held for at least 3 to 10 minutes. Once again, this depends on how much flow of Reiki energy the client needs. A standard treatment usually takes 45 minutes to 1 ½ hours.

How does a Reiki treatment feel?

The experience or feeling during a Reiki treatment is different from one client to another. However, all clients of a Reiki treatment will definitely experience a feeling of deep relaxation. In most cases, clients tend to drift off to sleep during the treatment.

Most clients who have already experienced a Reiki treatment claimed to have a glowing radiance surrounding and flowing through them. In addition, a state of well-being and peace is experienced given that the Reiki energy promotes letting go of all fear, anxiety, tension, or other negative feelings. Others claim to float outside their bodies while some claim to have mystical visions or experiences.

Once the treatment session ends, a client would surely feel refreshed and at the same time have a more balanced and positive outlook.

What does Reiki treat?

Reiki has a positive effect on almost all kinds of negative conditions and illness. These include minor physical conditions, such as bee stings, stomach aches, flu, and colds and major physical conditions, such as cancer, heart disease, and leukemia among others. Reiki also has the ability to relieve emotional and mental problems, including anxiety and depression.

Reiki can also reduce or eliminate side effects from regular medical treatments, including post-operative depression and pain and negative effects of chemotherapy. It can also improve one's healing rate as well as reduce the period of hospital confinement.

There are numerous cases wherein Reiki treatment has helped. In fact, some people who have gone through Reiki treatment sessions have claimed complete healing as confirmed from their medical tests before and after they have undergone Reiki treatment.

While Reiki can bring about miracles to some clients, this cannot be vouched. The true promise of a Reiki treatment is reduction of stress as well as improvement in an individual's psychological and physical condition.

To receive a Reiki treatment, does one need to stop seeing a psychologist or regular doctor?

An individual who wants to experience a Reiki treatment does not need to stop seeing his or her doctor. This is because Reiki can work in conjunction with regular psychological or medical treatments.

In fact, most Reiki practitioners would recommend seeing a licensed health care specialist in addition to undergoing Reiki treatment sessions, especially if the client has a psychological or medical condition.

Reiki can work with all other healing forms, including surgery, medications, alternative care methods, and psychological care.

Can anyone learn to do the Reiki?

Given that Reiki is a simple technique, more and more people regardless of age, gender, or nationality, are learning it. One does not need any prior experience with meditation, healing, or any type of training to learn the Reiki. This is because it is taught in a non-conventional manner where a teacher transfers the Reiki energy to the student through a process referred to as attunement. Once the student receives an attunement, he or she already has the ability to do the Reiki. The student can already place his or her hands to treat oneself or another individual as the healing Reiki energy automatically begins to flow.

Are children allowed to learn the Reiki?

Even children can learn the Reiki as long as they are old enough to understand the concepts of the Reiki system. It is also recommended for children to receive the Reiki.

How many levels are there in a Reiki training?

There are four levels in a Reiki training based on the Usui or Tibetan Reiki system. These include first, second, advanced, and Master levels.

How long will it take for one to learn the Reiki?

More often than not, Reiki centers that offer classes start on a weekend, specifically for beginners. The class usually takes one or two days. It is highly recommended to finish at least 6 to seven hours of a Reiki class. In addition, apart from the attunement, a student is also shown how to give treatments to oneself and to others as well as practice giving treatments during class.

What does Reiki attunement mean?

A Reiki attunement is the process wherein an individual receives the ability to provide Reiki treatments. During a Reiki class, a Reiki Master administers the attunement and touches the head, shoulders, and hands of the student while making use of one or more breathing techniques. The attunement energies then flow through the Reiki Master going to the student. Attunement energies are special energies, which are guided by the Higher Power. These energies also adjust through the energy pathways of the student, connecting him or her to the Reiki source.

During the attunement, the energetic aspect, which is guided by the Higher Power adjusts itself to become exactly what the student needs. Some students may have visions of spiritual beings or see colors during the attunement. Others may feel warmth in their hands. On the other hand, students undergoing an attunement may simply feel more relaxed without having an inner experience. In both cases, an attunement works.

Can an individual get more than one attunement?

An attunement lasts a lifetime; as such, when one receives as attunement, it will last his or her whole life. If one gets an additional attunement for the similar level, it will strengthen and refine the Reiki energy.

What is lineage?

Once an individual receives Reiki, he or she will be part of a succession of teachers, which leads to the founder of the Reiki system. For instance, if a teacher practices the Usui Reiki, the lineage would lead to Dr. Usui.

What can an individual expect or feel when giving a Reiki treatment?

When a practitioner gives a Reiki treatment, the Reiki energy flows through him or her prior to leaving the hands and flowing to the client. As such, the practitioner also receives a treatment. When the Reiki energy flows, the practitioner will feel uplifted and more relaxed. Some practitioners claim to have spiritual experiences when giving treatment. Others claim to receive insights about the client's needs, allowing them to heal in a deeper way.

Can a practitioner treat oneself?

Once a practitioner receives the attunement, he or she can treat oneself and others. This is one of Reiki's unique features as other types of healing or treatment do not allow an individual to treat oneself.

How does sending Reiki to others at a distance work?

During the second level of the Reiki training, a practitioner is given three symbols, which are empowered during the attunement. One of the three symbols include distant healing.

Reiki distance healing works by securing a picture of the individual whom the practitioner wants to send Reiki to. The practitioner may also write the individual's name on a paper; think of the person; or activate the distant symbol to send Reiki regardless of where the individual is located. There is no difference in the quality of Reiki healing a practitioner provides whether the client is near or hundreds of miles away. The Reiki energy will go directly to the client and treat him or her. Some practitioners also send Reiki to world leaders, especially during critical or crisis situations to help them.

Is Reiki treatment safe for pregnant women?

Given that the Reiki energy is guided by the Higher Power, it will know the client's condition and adjust as needed. Only positive and good things are provided during a Reiki treatment. As such, many women, even those who are pregnant receive Reiki treatments. Apart from providing great benefits to pregnant women, Reiki also treats the unborn child. Reiki is also used during child birth.

Is Reiki treatment safe for babies?

 Most babies who have received Reiki treatment love it. The Reiki energy adjusts to the needs of babies; therefore, parents do not need to worry about the treatment or energy being too strong.

Can Reiki also treat animals and plants?

Most animals that receive Reiki treatment seem to have an innate understanding of the Reiki as well as its benefits. Plants also have a positive response to Reiki as they grow healthier and stronger.

Does the Reiki treatment involve any side effects?

While people who receive the Reiki treatment feel uplifted and relaxed after a Reiki treatment, some individuals experience a "healing crisis." When an individual's vibration heightens, the toxins stored in the body are released into the blood stream, filtered by the kidneys and liver, and removed from the system. As a result, an individual may feel weak, or experience a stomach ache, or a headache. More often than not, practitioners recommend that the client experiencing these minor side effects drink more water, get more rest, and eat lighter meals. A huge part of the Reiki treatment is cleansing the body.

Can Reiki help groups of people during global crises?

One of the unique benefits of Reiki is that it is able encourage groups of people to do positive things even during challenging global situations. It is able to reduce the suffering of people across the globe.

How can an individual find a Reiki teacher who is right for him or her?

More often than not, Reiki Masters, practitioners, or teachers post advertisements in magazines, health food stores, book stores, and other places. When an individual finds a Reiki teacher, it is advisable to ask important questions to help in determining whether the said teacher is a good choice.

Some of the common questions to ask Reiki Masters, practitioners, or teachers include: how long have they been working with Reiki; what training have they undergone; how do they use Reiki personally; what is their lineage; how often do they teaches Reiki; what is covered in their classes; what qualifications are required in their Reiki training; how many hours of class time do they include; how much time is hands-on practice and instructional; what are their fees; does the class include a manual and certificate; and are they open to supporting students to become successful Reiki teachers or practitioners among others.

An individual should be aware of his or her feelings about the answers to his or her questions. A Reiki Master should be able to respond in a supportive, loving, and empowering manner. The individual should listen to his or her heart as the Reiki Master answers the questions.

How much is cost for each Reiki treatment?

A Reiki treatment generally costs around $25 to $100. The rate depends on the area as well as the country. On the other hand, some practitioners offer Reiki treatments for a donation or even free of charge.

Can an individual make Reiki a source of income?

If an individual puts his or her heart into Reiki, he or she can develop a Reiki practice while conducting classes. This is a fulfilling way that result in regular income.

Can an individual become "licensed" to practice and teach Reiki?

As of now, there are no licensing programs that any government provides to become a "licensed" Reiki practitioner. However, there are some Reiki centers that offer licensing programs for Reiki teachers.

Are Reiki treatments covered by insurance?

Some insurance companies cover Reiki treatments although most of them are just starting to recognize Reiki.

Conclusion

Reiki healing allows you to connect with the energies of the Universe and use it in a way that encourages the body to heal itself. It can be used to treat aches and pains, overcome allergies and headaches, and even heal chronic or painful diseases. The results depend heavily on your abilities and your mindset, as it is important to be receptive to the Reiki energies for them to result.

Often, the emotional and physical health problems that we struggle with stem from blocked energy channels in the body. Energy channels can be blocked after certain life circumstances or from being neglected. As you learn to encourage the flow of Universal energy through your body, you can promote overall health and wellness. You can stop at learning to heal yourself or you can continue our practice to strengthen your abilities and possibly heal others.

Hopefully, this book has been able to help provide the foundation for Reiki knowledge that you can build upon later. For the time being, however, you should know what you need to put your Reiki skills to work. The only thing left to do is practice! Your abilities will strengthen with time and as you become more aware of the way that the energies of the universe and your body affect you.

Best of luck!